D0728591

Linking the Strands of Language and Literacy

A RESOURCE MANUAL

Linking the Strands of Language and Literacy

A RESOURCE MANUAL

Candace L. Goldsworthy, PhD

With contributions by
Katie Lambert, MS

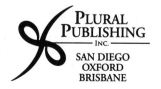

PLURAL
PUBLISHING
INC.
SAN DIEGO
OXFORD
BRISBANE

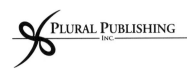

5521 Ruffin Road
San Diego, CA 92123

e-mail: info@pluralpublishing.com
Web site: http://www.pluralpublishing.com

49 Bath Street
Abingdon, Oxfordshire OX14 1EA
United Kingdom

Copyright © by Plural Publishing, Inc. 2010

Typeset in 11/13 Garamond by Flanagan's Publishing Services, Inc.
Printed in the United States of America by Bang Printing

All rights, including that of translation, reserved. No part of this publication may be
reproduced, stored in a retrieval system, or transmitted in any form or by any means,
electronic, mechanical, recording, or otherwise, including photocopying, recording,
taping, Web distribution, or information storage and retrieval systems without the
prior written consent of the publisher.

For permission to use material from this text, contact us by
Telephone: (866) 758-7251
Fax: (888) 758-7255
e-mail: permissions@pluralpublishing.com

*Every attempt has been made to contact the copyright holders for material originally
printed in another source. If any have been inadvertently overlooked, the publishers
will gladly make the necessary arrangements at the first opportunity.*

Library of Congress Cataloging-in-Publication Data

Goldsworthy, Candace L.
 Linking the strands of language and literacy : a resource manual / Candace L.
Goldsworthy ; with contributions by Katie Lambert.
       p. cm.
 Includes bibliographical references and index.
 ISBN-13: 978-1-59756-357-4 (alk. paper)
 ISBN-10: 1-59756-357-9 (alk. paper)
 1. Language acquisition. 2. Literacy. I. Lambert, Katie. II. Title.
 [DNLM: 1. Language Development. 2. Educational Status. 3. Language Disorders.
4. Speech-Language Pathology. WS 105.5.C8 G622L 2010]
 P118.G575 2010
 401'.93—dc22
                                                                    2009050887

Contents

Preface

I think I've always wanted to write this book—to simplify the murkiness that can exist when one considers working with the multivarious strands and levels inherent in a developing oral-written language system. Over the years as researchers and practitioners have contributed to our knowledge of language development, we have, at times, become confused with the myriad of models, categories, and labels. Perhaps because of, perhaps in spite of, the overwhelming influx of available language tests and materials, practitioners working with childhood language problems have become frustrated with targets, strategies, approaches, and programs. We are both blessed and haunted by the variations that exist in assessment tools for oral-written language. One identifies concepts to be worked on, another highlights parts of speech such as pronouns, adjectives, and prepositions. Still others zero in on syntactic constructions children should master at various ages. Thus, despite our increased knowledge of both normal and disordered language, those who must assess and remediate oral and written language problems too often are faced with the practical questions, "Where do I begin?" and "What should I work on next?"

Furthermore, after having supervised hundreds of student clinicians over my career as a university professor, I have been struck with the similarity in questions asked over the course of a semester's work. At the beginning of their Child Language Clinic, students are fearful about, well, everything from meeting the client, to what tests to use, to what materials to bring in, to what on earth they will do to fill a whole hour. At that juncture, I usually give the "everything will be fine" lecture, and everything usually is. Student clinicians then get through the first hurdles of assessing child language, targeting initial goals and objectives (standards and benchmarks), and selecting materials to use in therapy. For several weeks, all is well in clinic halls as student clinicians experiment with various materials, practice clinical techniques, and discuss their clients with their supervisors and with each other. Then crisis time! Invariably, about 6 to 8 weeks into a semester, back they come with "Oh, my gosh! It worked! The child got it! S/he is using the construction(s) I've been targeting since the beginning of the semester." When I try to assure them that this is the way it's supposed to work, they typically retort: "But I just got comfortable with what I was doing. What on earth am I going to do next?" And so it goes. They select more targets and materials, and practice another few weeks and it hits again. And so the roller-coaster of Child Language Clinic continues until the end of the semester. Usually by then I get to hear comments such as, "Wow! That was fun. I had no idea what I was doing some of the time but I got through it. I wish I could do it again because I know so much more now. If I'd only known *then* what I know *now*, I wouldn't have been so *scared*."

As beginning clinicians and many seasoned practitioners move through what seems like layers upon layers of language issues some of our clients present with, they face a number of relevant questions. "How do I know when to drop working on one language strand and move to another?" "When do I leave a strand such as listening skills to work on narrative skills?" "How do I add in the strand leading toward written language? How do I bridge *that* gap?"

I think I've always wanted to write this book because I've always loved child language-literacy. I've wanted to write this so beginning clinicians would have someplace to start and come back to time and time again to see what might be the next target to include in a child's instructional program. And I've wanted to write this for seasoned practitioners to check in from time to time to keep track of where they've been and what possibilities there are to include in child language-literacy instruction. Particularly now when the field of speech-language pathology has embraced the notion that language truly is on an oral-to-written continuum, it seems appropriate to include a range of oral language, reading, and written language goals together in one source.

This book is designed for beginning and seasoned speech-language pathologists and others in regular and special education who work with students demonstrating oral and written language problems. The intent of this book is to provide a resource of excellence, a schema of good practice. Wherever you are in your practice, you can use this book with a growing sense toward expertise. You may enter this book as a beginning clinician and move to a more advanced level, then move toward proficiency, to advanced proficiency, and finally to expert. As you use the suggested goals and materials, you will get more and more experience with the various language strands, and with more practice your skills will become automatic.

I've wanted a resource manual of child language-literacy instruction based on the way I "visualize" or think about child language-literacy. I have appreciated the view of the acquisition and development of language proposed by Dickinson and McCabe (1991) as a French braid. They wrote:

> The process of language acquisition can be thought of as being like a French braid rather than as a sequential process. Like a braid, language consists of multiple strands—phonology, semantics, syntax, discourse, reading, and writing—that are picked up at various times and woven in with the other strands to create a beautiful whole. (p. 1)

What a wonderful analogy! And what profession is better suited to assist in "braiding" than speech-language pathology? With a curriculum steeped in linguistics, child language acquisition and disorders, and numerous clinical hours in child language, the speech-language pathologist develops a keen sense of the underpinnings of language, of the oral-written language continuum. The speech-language pathologist is in a pivotal position to dissect language to identify what is occurring in a child's acquisition process that needs scaffolding to be able to move along the continuum. Using the French braid analogy, the speech-language pathologist joins the educational team equipped with background knowledge and experience to know which language strand is weak and what needs to be added in to strengthen the overall "braid." Because of their unique training, speech-language pathologists know how to assess discrete aspects of language, target instruction to strengthen those parts, and then to weave those discrete aspects into the bigger language domains, into the bigger picture, ultimately a client's oral-written language system.

As defined in Webster's dictionary (2002), one definition of strand is "any one of the threads, fibers, wires, etc. that are twisted together to form a length of string, rope, or cable; any of the individual bundles of thread or fiber so twisted together; any of the parts that are bound together to form a whole" (p. 626). The language-literacy continuum involves a number of strands developing separately and alongside each other, coming together to strengthen language-literacy acquisition until they merge onto a super highway of a fully developed oral-written language system. Like in the braid, the language-literacy strands represent what a child must develop to go from a simple to more complex language system, namely, listening skills to emergent oral language, to emergent written language including reading and writing. This resource reviews how the strands of language-literacy develop similarly, that is, the development of oral language, reading and writing strands evolve from whole to part and the development of each strengthens and reinforces the development of the other strands. It is not the purpose of this resource to train students in data collection. Please go to http://www.asha.org for references to this important topic, for instance, the article by Olswang and Bain (1994).

At the time of writing this book, some in our field are saying that we, as speech-language pathologists, can no longer work from the medical model dividing language into receptive and expressive components. Many are proposing that, if we work in the schools we must work with students' curriculum to support their work in the classroom. I could not agree more with this, but I think we must work on underlying weak structures, or language-literacy strands, to scaffold and merge into higher level language strands. After the language strands have been strengthened, working on the language of the curriculum is appropriate. Offering only language therapy related to school curriculum without remediating a compromised language foundation is tantamount to providing band-aid therapy.

This is an exciting time for the field of speech-language pathology. Our national organization, the American Speech-Language-Hearing Association (ASHA) is not asking speech-language pathologists to teach reading. Rather, and importantly, ASHA has asked practitioners to support literacy. The following is included among the guidelines for roles and responsibilities of speech-language pathologists in literacy by the American Speech, Language, and Hearing Association (2001):

> The practice of speech-language pathology involves: providing prevention, screening, consultation, assessment and diagnosis, treatment, intervention, management, counseling, and follow-up services for

disorders of . . . language (i.e., phonology, morphology, syntax, semantics, and pragmatic/social aspects of communication) including comprehension and expression in oral, written, graphic, and manual modalities; language processing; preliteracy and language-based literacy skills. (pp. 7–8)

At the same time, current testing methods allowing general education students to "wait to fail" before being identified as having learning disabilities are being challenged. Proposed changes in IDEA 2004 will allow local education agencies (LEAs) to use a pre-identification strategy known as response to intervention (RTI) in which at-risk students are taught key components of reading instruction, thereby possibly avoiding the need to be enrolled in special education. In an attempt to reduce misdiagnosis of students with learning disabilities (LD), dramatic changes appear in the 2004 Individuals with Disabilities Education Act (IDEA). In diagnosing leasrning disorders, a discrepancy criterion, in fact, is no longer necessary. The new act states:

. . . a local educational agency shall not be required to take into consideration whether a child has a severe discrepancy between achievement and intellectual ability in oral expression, listening comprehension, written expression, basic reading skill, reading comprehension, mathematical calculation, or mathematical reasoning (614,h,6,A).

These changes will allow LEAs to measure a student's responses to scientific, research-based intervention as a part of the evaluation procedures inherent in RTI, the focus of which is on providing early effective instruction for students experiencing difficulties in learning to read. The components of the RTI were named in the Put Reading First program that identified the following five key components as the essential building blocks of reading: phonemic awareness, phonics instruction, vocabulary development, fluency and text comprehension.

Across the country speech-language pathologists are taking leadership roles in supporting literacy. Historically, their training in language acquisition and disorders, linguistics and phonetics, coupled with many hours of clinical experience, positions the speech-language pathologist as key to working most directly with children and adolescents with developmental language problems. This resource manual of child language intervention is intended to fortify today's practitioners in those leadership roles by providing a review of the oral-written language continuum with possible targets and suggested materials.

This resource is not intended to teach the underlying theory of language disorders. Rather, the purpose of this volume is to bring together suggested targets and materials in selected oral-written language areas. Because the intent of this book is to be a resource for practitioners working with children and adolescents with developing language-literacy and with disordered/delayed language-literacy, materials have been brought together under chapter headings indicating each language-literacy strand. Three primary sources were considered in selecting the targeted strands: first, a background in speech-language pathology; second, the Position Statement present by the American Speech-Language Hearing Association (2001) on the Roles and Responsibilities of Speech-Language Pathologists With Respect to Reading and Writing in Children and Adolescents; and third, the recommendations by the National Reading Panel (2004). The chapters in this resource include:

1. Overview of the strands of language and literacy
2. Play
3. Listening skills
4. Early oral-written language: the rationale
5. Linking the strands of oral-written language: The how-tos
6. Oral narration outlines and language literacy activities
7. Companion CD

In each chapter, selected teaching targets are outlined followed by sample materials available in the field. I have compiled materials in the clinics where I work with students and clients. Materials are described so that a practitioner in another part of the country who does not have access to the exact material described, will be able to find or compile similar materials in their clinical/ teaching site.

Acknowledgments

Dr. Goldsworthy wishes to acknowledge the graduate student clinicians and fellow practitioners who have asked the questions, the colleagues who have listened and helped arrive at solutions, and the children with language problems who taught us all.

Mrs. Lambert would like to thank her husband and biggest fan, Tait, her parents, Thomas and Belinda Hussey, who have always believed in her; Papa and Gram, Dr. Goldsworthy and the professors in the Speech-Language Pathology and Audiology Department at California State University, Sacramento, and the professional staff of Speech Language Learning Associates for the knowledge and encouragement of future clinicians to find their places in this great field.

Chapter 1

Overview of the Strands of Language and Literacy

As mentioned in the Preface, the materials in this resource manual have been arranged according to language strands, with various strands representing the levels a child must pass through to transition from early oral language skills to higher written language skills. A client on your caseload may need to have targets selected from the beginning strand(s), such as listening skills, and then proceed up through the various higher language strands. Or, a client may be struggling with targets selected somewhere in the middle of the language strands, for example, early reading and writing, and may need to go back to earlier language levels, such as phonological awareness, then move back up to reading targets. What clinicians, new or experienced, must keep in mind, and what will be reiterated throughout this manual, is the dynamic, fluid nature of the language acquisition process. Language is not acquired in a discrete stairstep fashion as many textbooks and therapy sources would have you think. Those presentations are to help us understand the many levels of language acquisition, which constitute the *science* of understanding language acquisition. The *art* of understanding language acquisition is being ever vigilant as to where the client currently is on the oral-written language continuum. The *art* is in knowing that, although the client may be demonstrating growth in one of the language strands, she or he may still need to strengthen a strand she or he has already passed through, as well as stay vigilant to emerging clues that the client may be moving toward another strand.

Child language is steeped in developmental charts. For instance, we know what sounds children usually acquire at what times in their development. Likewise, we know when the typically developing child acquires various semantic relations, vocabulary, syntactic constructions and transformations, and what is pragmatically appropriate in the use of language at various age levels. Typically, in child language therapy, one language domain is targeted at a time, namely phonology, semantics, syntax, *or* social-pragmatics. Said differently, at any given time, the focus of language therapy may be content (meaning), form (phonology or syntax-morphology), or use (pragmatics). In an effort to try to simplify child language therapy through a strands approach, the resource manual's approach is contrasted with the traditional child language therapy approach. One of the goal attack strategies in child language therapy (see McCauley & Fey, 2006) is to implement a "vertical approach strategy," working with one goal at a time. The strands approach promotes working more on a "horizontal attack strategy," working on more than one goal at a time, as well as working on more than one strand at a time. Stated differently, a strands approach promotes working on, perhaps, an oral language goal as well as on a printed language goal such as reading, and a written goal to increase the client's ability to write words or phrases. Working on these goals simultaneously helps to meld them—to strengthen each because of growth in the other—each scaffolding the other.

Many students and seasoned practitioners of child language therapy select targets to include in therapy based on what the used assessment tools dictate. How many times have I read student reports and lesson plans identifying pronouns "he," "she," and "it," to be the focus of therapy—for 12 weeks! The client then demonstrates that she or he can produce "he" or "she" within the therapy session but not outside the therapy room. How can we facilitate the acquisition of a *linguistic system*? Not just language parts! As I pointed out in *Developmental Reading Disabilities: A Language-Based Treatment Approach* (2003), rather than identifying and treating isolated deficit areas in a child's oral language system, we need to examine the impact this deficit may have on the child's developing reading comprehension and written language system. With the exception of very young children, or children with extremely delayed language systems, why are we targeting oral language isolated from written language? By opening our kaleidoscope to a bigger picture, wouldn't our language therapy be far more effective if we examined the impact that oral language problems have on the bigger picture, that is, the child's oral-written language system? We can identify specific words or parts of speech, for instance, "he" and "she" as noted above, and teach a child to understand and use only these two pronouns or, far better, submerge this child in pronouns in general both in oral language and through print (i.e., read books with many pronouns as examplars, not just "he" and "she").

For some time, my concern has been that in language therapy we work on the language parts and not the whole—not the gestalt. A language strands approach works to remedy this by braiding the strands, bringing in more than one strand at a time, and working across modalities—talking, reading, and writing.

As adults, it is impossible for us to recall how the strands of our "language braid" gradually became intertwined to the point that we possessed an evolved oral-written language system. There are many analogies to help remind us how this might work. Learning to play a sport such as golf provides a rich example of how many features of a game have to be practiced and skills learned to "get it" to actually say you can play the sport. Novice golfers are all too familiar with learning the many skills that finally come together to play the game: learning about long and short games; woods and irons; the differences between putting, chipping, and pitching, to name just a few. While taking lessons and during early outings on the golf course, the novice player moves between feeling frustrated with hitting too short and putting too long, hitting balls that go too far to the right or the left, to feeling elated when that little white ball actually goes where the golfer intended.

Before further describing a strands approach to language-literacy, I have two personal analogies to further illustrate how a skill may need to be "dissected" for one to learn it or to improve something. My first analogy is that of relearning, as an adult, how to play the piano, and my second involves learning how to oil paint.

First, the piano. A few years ago I could barely read the music to play some notes with my right hand. I had no recollection of how to read music for the left hand. Slowly, with a very patient instructor and a lot of practice, I learned where to place my fingers on the keyboard, first with the right hand alone and then the left hand alone. Then I practiced exercises to help me move up and down the keyboard faster, while also continuing to practice "reading" the music. I gradually became more fluent in reading music with both hands simultaneously but still needed to repeat and add in more "drill work" at earlier levels to scaffold my reading the music. During the course of my piano lessons, I am frequently amazed that my piano instructor gives me new music each week to learn something different about playing the instrument.

In child language, we have been trained over the years that our clients should perform at the 80% accuracy level twice in a row (over at least two sessions) to prove they have mastered the targeted goal(s). So, as practitioners, we isolate a target, a pronoun, an adjective, a passive transformation, and so forth, and we teach it, probe for it, then measure the use of it. We expect that clients have "mastered" this if they perform at the 80% accuracy level twice in a row. In piano lessons, I have not reached 80% performance level on most songs! *Yet*, my piano instructor rarely has me repeat a piece. Rather, I am introduced to one or two new pieces per week to practice and perform during the next week's lesson. I suspect the reason for this is each new lesson has helped me learn one or another aspect of piano playing (reading the music, moving up and down the keyboard, timing, when to use the pedal, how loud or soft to play). Each aspect is scaffolding on the other. I attempt to learn one aspect through practicing one piece one week and another aspect on another piece the next. And so it goes, week by week, with each aspect scaffolding and supporting the other as I get stronger, as the elements of playing the piano come together for me. Lesson after lesson, strand after strand is laid down forming the foundation I need to move toward some sort of gestalt of piano playing. When I asked my piano instructor about this, she reinforced the idea of scaffolding and added an interesting point—by continuing to move me forward on a weekly basis, we "keep it fresh." In other words, rather than have me practice one piece of music focusing on one aspect of piano playing week after week, and ultimately becoming weary of the piece and unmotivated to practice, new material focusing on various aspects is "keeping it fresh" and keeps me motivated to continue. In child language therapy, we can keep it fresh by introducing new strands while continuing to focus on ones we have already targeted.

To further indulge my right hemisphere, I am now learning how to oil paint. Again, I have been fortunate to have selected incredibly talented instructors who have taught me to work on one part of the painting at a time, stand back to view the painting, and then to reflect on how this part now fits the gestalt, or the whole painting. Then they encourage me to work on another part of the painting and again to stand back and think about the effect this part has on the rest of the painting. I have learned what they mean by "move around the canvas/painting," working on one area, then another, and returning to the previous area to add to it. One of my instructors, internationally known Susan Sarback of Fair Oaks, California, explained the importance of thinking of the gestalt:

> Most people tend to isolate colors . . . this is red and this is blue, but if you look at music you realize quickly that one note taken out of a song is nothing. It's only its relationship to other notes that makes a song. And many songs can have the same notes, but the sound is totally different. It's the same with colors. (by permission of the author, 2008)

In her work on the natural human learning process, Smilkstein (2002) explained that from an early age, cognitively intact humans possess innate learning processes making it possible for them to learn complex, abstract skills and ideas. She maintains that the human brain is a powerful natural learning organ because it has a natural learning process, innate logic, is a natural problem-solver and pattern-seeker, and is internally motivated. Smilkstein's (2003) work described six stages in the natural human learning process. She summarized these as follows:

Stage 1: Motivation involves responding to a stimulus in the environment, not knowing how it works but just being interested/curious in it.

Stage 2: Beginning practice involves a lot of trial and error and practice; asking for help; more practice; making mistakes; more practice.

Stage 3: Advanced practice involves more practice and having some successes; asking questions, and growing confidence and skill.

Stage 4: Skillfulness involves more practice; beginning to do something your own way with increased confidence; able to share your knowledge.

Stage 5: Refinement involves increased improvement and learning new methods; you are validated by others; new skill becoming a habit.

Stage 6: Mastery involves broader application of skill; you can teach it to others.

As Smilkstein pointed out, the six stages occur naturally in cognitively intact human beings and a vital component in the process is practice. It would seem that children with language-learning issues would need to have methods, materials, and guidance to traverse these same six stages in their travels to communicate through oral and written language. Our job as speech-language pathologists working with these children would be to select targets and introduce remediation, ever sensitive to the natural stages of the human learning process described above. Simple enough, right? But not so simple when we consider an intriguing description of what happens when children don't practice one critical aspect of language acquisition, namely, listening. Johnston (2006) pointed out that:

> Children normally develop selective listening skills in late infancy, but lags in neural maturation, perceptual deficits, or language delays may hinder this achievement. Children who don't talk get much less practice in listening. If they find the auditory world confusing they may even choose not to listen. (p. 93)

Children with language-learning problems don't get much practice with various skills and, in fact, may choose to not engage in them during their development. As Smilkstein (2003) noted that when it comes to the important natural human learning process, "use it or lose it" takes on new meaning. Dendrites grow for what is practiced, while the learner's brain is busy at work constructing new neural networks specific for each new object of learning, and when not used, dendrites and neurons are pruned for "ecological efficiency." Furthermore, Smilkstein explained that, like twigs on trees, dendrites grow off what is already there. New skills and concepts, therefore, are developed through a connection with the learner's prior knowledge or experience.

To be more specific about how strands of language-literacy therapy might work, because of my work in oral and written literacy over the years, I have come to believe more and more in introducing clients to various aspects of language such as increasing vocabulary or expanding the length and complexity of syntactic utterances through oral *and* written language. I typically introduce something through implicit teaching and move to explicit teaching. In implicit teaching, I am simply introducing a client to certain targets through play therapy or a book or conversation about some topic. When the client shows an interest in the topic, I move to explicit teaching wherein I make the target more readily apparent, that is to say, make it stand out as key. Through practicing the target(s), the client increases exposure to receptively understanding the target and expressively producing it/them. Rather than "hold out" for 80% accuracy on established targets, I move up to the next targets in those strands *as well as review* targets already included on that strand(s). Much like Hodson and Paden's (1991) cycles approach to phonological processes, the basic tenets include focusing on perception and production following a sequence of activities. In the case of phonological processes, the sequence of activities include: auditory bombardment, production practice, probes to check stimulability, and then more auditory bombardment. In their approach, Hodson and Paden suggest that certain target phonemes such as /sp/ and /st/ are selected *to represent* the target phonological pattern of cluster reduction. A cycle is complete when all patterns have been treated but not necessarily remediated. The remaining patterns are recycled. Mastery is not a criterion for moving to the next treatment target.

In the current resource, after play and early listening skills, the intent of this work is to promote a cycles approach to language therapy in which various exemplars are selected to represent various language areas. To that end, three more strands have been included in this resource. Because the critical social pragmatic communication has been covered in detail in a number of other sources, it has not been included in this book. Although the following list is included for the reader's organization, a truer picture of the intent of this manual are braided strands—these help us visualize the dynamic nature of weaving in play with early listening skills, which overlap and weave into early phonological processing of receptive and expressive language, and then meld into early reading and writing (Figure 1–1). Included in this source:

Chapter 2: Play

Chapter 3: Listening Skills

Chapter 4: Early Oral-Written Language: The Rationale

Chapter 5: Linking the Strands of Oral-Written Language: The How Tos

Chapter 6: Oral Narration Outlines and Language Literacy Activities by Katie R. Lambert, MS, with accompanying CD of downloadable materials.

Language Ladder: Where to Begin Teaching/Remediating

Phonological Awareness
Word level
Syllable level
Phoneme level

Expressive/Oral Language
Verbal repetition
Oral vocabulary
Syntax/morphology
Oral narrative skills: personal
  and fictional narrative
Multiple meaning words
Analogic thinking

Receptive Language
Simple receptive language
Basic concepts
Categorization
Listening comprehension

Central Auditory Processing
Auditory discrimination
Auditory temporal pattern recognition
Auditory figure-ground selection
Auditory selective attention
Auditory memory
Auditory integration

Figure 1–1. The language ladder. Copyright Candace Goldsworthy 2010.

Written Language
Emergent skills (draw
  print, patterns)
Early words &
  word families
Words from books
Written narratives
Written syntax/
  morphology
Spelling
Capitalization/
  punctuation
Writing fluency
Proofing

Reading
Emergent skills (print, book, story
  knowledge)
Phonological awareness
Sound symbol association (word
  attack/decoding)
Letter-word identification
Word families
Reading comprehension
Reading fluency: accuracy, rate,
  prosody

Word Retrieval
Word finding/retrieval
Word finding/retrieval in
  discourse

Chapter 2

Play

*E*ntire books have been written on children's play. And with the huge surge of interest in children on the autism spectrum even more books have surfaced covering a multitude of invaluable information on attachment theory, joint attention, and the expansion of play skills. The purpose of including this important topic here is twofold: first to remind ourselves that we may, in fact, need to begin with or move back to this important strand with children. I remind my child language clinicians that children don't necessarily come into our clinics ready to sit at tables and be assessed with language assessment tools. Likewise, they may be far from being ready to sit at a small table and cooperate readily with efforts to engage them in direct language therapy. Too often, in our zeal to increase a child's language system, we impose table sitting and structured language activities on some children who are just not ready to engage with us at that level. Listen to what your children ask of you during therapy sessions. They may be 7, 8, or 9 years old but when a child asks "are you going to play with me?" with the trucks, blocks, or whatever the child chooses to play with, you need to listen. A child who wants you to get down and play with him or her needs to have this strand added into or back into the language session. The information in this chapter is presented under the following questions:

- How does children's play develop?
- What do children talk about?
- What are various types of children's play?
- What kind of concepts do young children acquire?
- What are specific word types and words to emphasize at various MLUs?
- What are some techniques to use in early phases of child language therapy?

How Does Children's Play Develop?

To help the student clinician and to briefly review play for the practicing/seasoned clinician, I have chosen to integrate four views or descriptions of play. It would seem helpful to introduce this strand with a brief review of the more traditional view of play's evolution as it relates to developmental growth from infancy to middle childhood. An excellent source for this review by Fernie (2000) summarizes three stages of play: (a) sensorimotor, (b) pretend/sociodramatic, and (c) play with games and rules.

Beginning with *sensorimotor play*, infants experiment with bodily sensation and motor movements through trial-and-error actions on them. With practice, infants and toddlers pull and push objects, move them around, and then eventually crawl after them. In sensorimotor play, infants and toddlers explore with bodily sensations and motor movements with objects and people. They like to roll balls, stack objects, put objects in containers and take them back out, knock things down, and enjoy toys that make noise such as rattles and bells. As they develop, young children discover that you can do more than one thing to objects. So, for instance, you can roll, kick, throw, and retrieve balls. You can knock blocks or boxes down and stack them back up to be knocked down again. You can stack boxes on top of each other and next to each other. At 9 months, the infant applies similar actions to most objects but by 12 months she or he shakes a rattle and rolls or kicks a ball. Two-year-olds move into experimenting with familiar objects such as brushing their hair or drinking from a cup. By 2½ years, the toddler stirs an imaginary drink and now offers it to someone else to drink.

Three-year-olds engage in pretend or *sociodramatic play* where they take on roles of familiar people in familiar daily life scripts they've witnessed such as eating. When they are 4 and 5 years old, children continue their pretend play with elaborated language scripts, often assigning roles to each other with "rules" that will be followed by the players (e.g., "you need to run away and hide this time and I'll stay right here"). The inclusion of rules in earlier play leads the way naturally to what the typically developing 5-year-old engages in when she or he becomes interested in *games with rules*. Game play is far more organized and involves children playing together in more logical and socialized ways, for example, with cards or game boards. Two Internet sources the reader may wish to access for more information in this area include: http://www .kidsource and http://www.nncc.org/curriculum. Both are cited in the References.

What Do Children Talk About?

Westby (2000) described the kind of play during the sensorimotor period as *presymbolic* occurring between 13 and 17 months of age in typically developing children. The kind of communication that accompanies this level includes context-dependent single words such as naming things (e.g., "doggie") when handing a stuffed animal to the adult. The kind of communication typical of this kind of play includes:

- interactions of requests ("gimme")
- commands ("mine")
- protests ("no")
- labeling ("car," "book")
- and greetings ("Hi," "Bye")

Westby referred to the beginning of the *symbolic phase* as *symbolic level I*, typically occurring between 17 and 19 months. During this time, children engage in familiar, everyday activities accompanied by short isolated schemas that are single pretend actions. As such, the child can pretend to engage in activities such as eating, sleeping, or drinking from an empty cup. Because this is the beginning of true verbal communication, the child interacts verbally with the adult through requesting and commanding using words that now represent relations between and among objects, that is, represent *semantic relations* such as recurrence: "more;" existence: "here;" rejection: "no," agents: "mommy," "daddy," doggie;" objects: "car," and actions: "eat."

Westby described the typically developing 19- to 22-month-old child as being in *symbolic level II* in which he or she acts on dolls or stuffed animals performing pretend actions on more than one object or person. More pretend play now involves short, isolated schema combinations such as holding the baby doll and covering it with a blanket, and the beginning of word combinations, including the following semantic relations: agent-action, agent-object, attributive, dative, action-locative, and possessive. During *symbolic level III*, which Westby described as occurring in typically developing children around 2 years of age, single schemas about daily experiences are elaborated with more details added into the play, such as stirring pretend food in a pan and placing the pan on the toy stove. There is an emergence of role reversing in play where the child wants to be you and asks you to be him or her. Language includes increasingly more comments and the child uses phrases and short sentences including the emergence of morphological endings such as plural /s/ ("cars"), marking present progressive verbs with –ing ("running"), and marking possessives with /s/ "(mommy's"). Westby maintained that, by 2½ years at *symbolic level IV*, the typically developing child is now involved in play where themes represent less frequently personal experienced events, such as going to the doctor or shopping at a store. Now the child is able to reverse roles with the adult, such as "I'll be the kid and you be the doctor," and language continues to expand primarily through ever-increasing use of question forms.

During *symbolic level V*, which Westby noted occurs in typically developing children around 3 years, children are able to modify outcomes of play scenarios. If "dad" went to the store to shop last week, "mom" may go this week. Episode sequences now become more involved and detailed such as the child cooks the food, serves it to others, clears the table, and washes the dishes. The child now reports, predicts, and narrates or tells the story as it evolves. The language that accompanies this expanded play now includes more past ("we went shopping") and future ("Daddy will be here") tenses. Westby's *symbolic level VI*, occurring between 3 and 3½ years, sees typically developing children carrying out pretend play with toys such as farms, barns, doll houses, and so forth with events being re-enacted where the child was not an active participant, for example, she or he now plays the firefighter, policeman, Batman, Spiderman, or Power Ranger. The child now assigns roles to other players, uses props, and "talks" for dolls or puppets. She or he now takes on and assigns multiple roles, for example, "I'll be the doctor and the nurse and you be the mom and the sick kid." She or he now expresses thoughts and feelings of the doll and is capable of changing her or his speech depending on which part she or he is taking in the play drama. Language now includes far more descriptive vocabulary in general including shapes, colors, sizes, and so forth. and the child now uses metacommunicative strategies (e.g., "He said . . . "). In Westby's *symbolic level VII*, typically occurring between 3½ to 4 years of age, the child and stuffed animal/doll continue to have multiple roles with the child now hypothesizing "What would happen if?" In *symbolic level VIII* at 5 years of age, themes of play become highly imaginative with many details acted out and discussed. The child now integrates scripts from previous play scenarios into new ones such as being the doctor, nurse, mom and sick kid in the jungle or outer space. The child can now plan ahead and gathers needed props for the scenes and scripts with themes that are now goal-directed. Language now includes relational terms (then, next, first, last, when, while, before, after). See Table 1–1 for a quick reference of Westby's play levels.

Just one of many examples of how this expanded play evolves comes from my work with 4-year-old Annie. One day Annie explained that her brother, Lucas, apparently ate too much broccoli one evening and complained later about an upset stomach. This led the way to reenactment during our therapy sessions, first with Annie telling about what happened, to telling me she would be "Dr. Seuss," and I would be Annie's mom. Our play reenactment started with the use of old cell phones and "mom" calling "Dr. Seuss" to complain that "Jared" (Annie's next door neighbor) was sick and needed to see a doctor. At first, play ended with this call. Annie simply put the phone down and walked away from the play scene. As ideas expanded surrounding this real-life scenario, coupled with her expanding linguistic repertoire, the play soon included the initiating call between Dr. Seuss and mom, a visit to the doctor's office and now adds props, the doctor bag with play utensils. Soon after, the scenario included all these plus lining up two chairs to represent our "car" as we drove mom, Lucas, Annie, and Jared to the doctor. Eventually, this play evolved into all of the above plus Annie picking up paper and pencil and jotting something, possibly a bill from the doctor or a prescription for the family to pick up medication for poor Jared. Simply put, Annie led the way as children usually will do with an ever vigilant adult there to add the appropriate props and ever expanding language to mirror the play scenario.

Table 2–1. Summary of Westby's (2000) Description of Play Development

Age	Phase	Typical Play	Corresponding Communication	Examples
13–17 mos.	Presymbolic	Context dependent	Single words	*Request:* "gimme" *Command:* "mine" *Label:* "car" *Protest:* "no" *Greeting:* "hi, bye"
17–19 mos.	Symbolic I	Single pretend actions representing familiar everyday activities such as eating, sleeping, drinking from cup	Beginning of true verbal communication using single words coding functional and semantic relations	*Recurrence:* "more" referring to "more cookie" *Rejection:* "no" referring to "don't want" *Agent:* "daddy" referring to daddy is doing something; *Existence:* "here" referring to "here's the cat" *Object:* "car" referring to what we're playing with *Denial:* "no" referring to "not me!"
19–22 mos.	Symbolic II	More pretend play with short isolated schema using props such as dolls or stuffed animals	Beginning of word combinations to code semantic relations	*Action-object:* "kick ball" *Possessive:* "mommy purse" *Agent-action:* "baby eat" *Attributive:* "pretty bunny" *Action-location:* "put there"

Age	Phase	Typical Play	Corresponding Communication	Examples
2 years	Symbolic III	More elaborated schemas about daily experiences such as eating and cooking; beginning to reverse roles; one day is mommy and next day is baby	Uses phrases and short sentences	"I want egg," "give me more," "cook red egg." Begins to mark plurals with /s/ ("cats"); present progressive verbs ("walking, running"); and possessives with /s/ ("mommy's"); makes comments about what she or he is doing ("eat cookie") and what other object does ("doggie walk")
2½ years	Symbolic IV	Themes about less personal events such as doctor visits; shopping for food	Reverses roles: "I'm daddy today and you're mommy," then "I'm mommy and you be the daddy"	Longer sentences; more question forms
3 years	Symbolic V	Modifies play scenario and outcomes; if daddy went shopping last week, mommy goes this week	More detailed episodes; more sequences of events; child cooks the food, serves it to others, clears the table, and washes the dishes	Begins to report, predict, narrate the story including past and future events

continues

17

Table 2–1. *continued*

Age	Phase	Typical Play	Corresponding Communication	Examples
3–3½ years	Symbolic VI	Pretend play with toys such as farms, barns, doll houses, etc.	Assigns multiple roles: "I'll be the doctor and the nurse and you be the mom and the sick kid. Involves roles she or he has not been before such as Superman, Spiderman or Power Ranger. Dolls or puppets changing speech depending on role taken	Far more descriptive vocabulary including shapes, colors, sizes, etc. and metacommunicative strategies such as "He said." "She said." Expresses thoughts and feelings of the doll or stuffed animal and can change his or her speech depending on which role he or she is taking.
3½–4 years	Symbolic VII	More pretend play	Can hypothesize	"What would happen if the fireman fell from the roof?"
5 years	Symbolic VIII	Themes of play become highly imaginative. Plans ahead and gathers props. Now themes are goal-directed	More details are acted out and discussed	Child now integrates scripts from previous play scenarios into new ones. Sequence/connecting words used: "then, next, first, last, when, while, before, after"

What Are Various Types of Children's Play?

The above example of Annie and Dr. Seuss provides one example of a kind of play (this time dramatic play) as a reenactment of a real life situation or event in this little girl's life and the expanding language that accompanied it. Children engage in several types of play and it is important for the adult interacting with them to be cognizant of what type of play the child is focused on at that point in time. The following discussion summarizes various types of children's play presented at http://www.nncc.org/Curriculum/better.play.html.

Quiet Play: encouraged through use of picture books, string beads, puzzles, pegboards, play with dolls, trucks, and so forth and coloring with markers or crayons.

Creative Play: painting, drawing, music, dancing, play dough, sand, collage, use of imagination, and problem solving.

Active Play: can be stimulated by use of balls, push-pull toys, sand and water play, musical instruments, bean bag toss, dress up clothes, cars and trucks as well as outside activities such as running, climbing trees, and so forth.

Cooperative Play: involves more than one person such as games, tag, dolls with doll house, block building, and hide and seek.

Dramatic Play: also referred to as social play, where children experiment with various life roles such as being a firefighter, mom, dad, teacher, farmer, or doctor. These episodes typically mirror their life experiences and these play scenarios will grow in depth as the child's cognitive-linguistic abilities are strengthened. As a language therapist, this kind of play lends itself to the greatest degree of language expansion but, once again, we must remember to follow the child's lead.

Manipulative Play: play that involves use of hands, muscles, eyes. Puzzles, crayons, pencils, painting, cutting with scissors, string beads, using tools, building with blocks, dolls, and trucks.

What Kind of Concepts
Do Young Children Acquire?

In planning relevant language therapy, we need to consider the typical concepts young children generally consider during the early years. What do they typically *want* to talk about? I can think of no greater reference for this topic than *The New Language of Toys* (Schwartz & Miller, 1996). I routinely require this as the textbook for a Methods course for Child Language Disorders.

In an informative online source for child's play, National Network for Child Care, cited above, the following suggestions were presented as appropriate toys for children's play. As pointed out in this source "there is no all-inclusive list of toys or the ways that children play with them." The network suggested the following five categories to consider when grouping toys for children.

■ **Toys for Physical Development:** wagons to steer and coast; brooms and shovels; small, but strong garden tools; balls; planks; jump ropes; scooters and tricycles; boxes, ladders, and boards; and puzzles.

■ **Toys for Sense Development** (touching, hearing, seeing, smelling, or tasting): water toys, bubble pipes, musical instruments, toy piano, xylophones, sand toys, pegboards, large wooden beads and string, puzzles.

■ **Toys for Creative Work:** Play-Doh or crayons and paints, colored paper, children's safety scissors, paste.

■ **Toys for Make Believe and Social Development:** dolls with washable clothes, adult "dress-up" clothes, cars and airplanes, broom sweeper, mop, dishes, play-store toys.

■ **Toys to Be Used for Building:** blocks, boards, boxes.

The network source cited above also looked at children's toys and developing concepts at the various ages, which are briefly summarized here.

■ **Child's Age Level: 0–18 Months.**
Children learn about *spatial relationships, shapes, and sizes* through nested cups and boxes, blocks, large puzzles, plas-

tic containers of various sizes. Their *cognitive skills* grow through pictured and rhyming books, and musical toys.

■ **Child's Age Level: 18 Months–3 Years.**
Symbolic representation is enhanced through playing with simple dress-up clothes, stuffed animals, dolls, and tea sets. *Language* continues to grow through use of more picture books, children's magazines and stories on tapes.

■ **Child's Age Level: 3–6 Years.**
Social and intellectual growth continues through, among others, more dress-up clothes, bathing and feeding dolls, store-keeping toys, toy phones, housekeeping toys, toy soldiers, dolls for dressing, and large puzzles. Increased *problem solving* can result from use of play sets such as the farmhouse, small trucks, cars, planes, and boats; beads, blocks, peg boards, simple construction sets, and car sets, housekeeping toys, trains, and race cars. *Form and spatial relationships* can be facilitated through use of simple puzzles, plastic measuring cups, and many outdoor toys. *Creativity* can grow through use of crayons, scissors, clay, paper, paste, and rhythm instruments. And the continued use of books will encourage continued language growth.

What Are Specific Word Types and Words to Emphasize at Various MLUs?

For an excellent source on how to calculate a child's mean length of utterance (MLU) the reader is referred to Hedge and Pomaville's (2008) assessment text. Their Language Assessment Protocol 6: Task-Specific Assessment Protocol for Grammatic Morphemes is presented in Figure 2–1. Although a bit time-consuming, MLU calculation and enhancement has been the way of language therapy in young children for years. I am amazed to hear that, in various parts of the country, language sampling and the calculation of MLU is going by the wayside. Stated simply, this has been the heart of language assessment in young children, and in many cases, it is the only measurement available to us because that's all the child is giving us.

Child's Name _____ DOB _____ Date _____

Clinician _____

Sample only the features that the child did not produce in his or her conversation with you (language sampling). Change words as needed, to suit the child's ethnocultural background. Add additional words within each category. Score a missing feature as incorrect.

Morpheme	Example	Correct	Incorrect
Present Progressive *ing*	He is *eating*.		
	She is *smiling*.		
	It is *jumping*.		
	They are *running*.		
	The cat is *sleeping*.		
	The boy is *reading*.		
	The girl is *riding* the horse.		
Regular Plural (*s, z, vz, əz*)	Two *cats*. (*s*)		
	I see two *cups*. (*s*)		
	They are two *dogs*. (*z*)		
	My *shoes* are white. (*z*)		
	Leaves are green. (*vz*)		
	I see *wolves*. (*vz*)		
	You have two *boxes*. (*əz*)		
	I see two *houses*. (*əz*)		
Irregular Plural	I see two *women*.		
	I have two *feet*.		
	I see three *mice*.		
	They are all *men*.		
	Many *children* come to my school.		
	I have many *teeth*.		

Figure 2–1. *Task-Specific Assessment Protocol for Grammatic Morphemes (From Assessment of Communication Disorders in Children: Resources and Protocols by M. N. Hegde and Frances Pomaville. Copyright © 2008 Plural Publishing, Inc. All rights reserved. Used with permission.)* continues

Morpheme	Example	Correct	Incorrect
Possessive (s, z, əz)	It is the *cat's* bowl. (s)		
	Elephant's trunk is long. (s)		
	It is my *Mommy's* bag. (z)		
	It is the *boy's* balloon. (z)		
	Santa Clause's *elves.* (əz)		
	It is the *horse's* tail. (əz)		
Prepositions (in, on, under, behind)	Car is *in* the bucket.		
	Pencil is *in* the mug.		
	The ball is *on* the table.		
	The book is *on* the floor.		
	The doll is *under* the table.		
	The coin is *under* the cup.		
	The book is *behind* the ball.		
	The cat is *behind* the box.		
Pronouns (she, he, it, they)	*She* bakes cookies.		
	She rides a bike.		
	He reads a book.		
	He eats a sandwich.		
	It moves slowly.		
	It licks its paw.		
	They are big trees.		
	They are eating apples.		
Conjunctions (and, but, because)	These are spoons *and* forks.		
	These are cups *and* plates.		
	She wants to paint, *but* there is no paint.		
	She wants to eat, *but* there is no food.		
	He is sleeping *because* he is tired.		
	She is eating *because* she is hungry.		

Figure 2–1. continues

Morpheme	Example	Correct	Incorrect
Irregular Past Tense	I ate the candy you gave me.		
	The pencil fell from your hand.		
	I went to school yesterday.		
	This car is broke.		
Regular Past Tense (*t, d, ted, ded,*)	Mom baked cookies. (*t*)		
	She talked on phone. (*t*)		
	You moved the chair. (*d*)		
	I closed the door. (*d*)		
	I painted on this paper. (*ted*)		
	I counted to 10. (*ted*)		
	You folded the paper. (*ded*)		
	You bended your finger. (*ded*)		
Articles (*a, the*)	I see *a* dog.		
	That is *a* chair.		
	The ant is small.		
	The elephant is big.		
Auxiliary (*is, was, are, were*)	The girl *is* talking on the phone.		
	The boy *is* kicking the ball.		
	Yesterday, Daddy *was* working in his office.		
	Yesterday, I *was* playing with my brother.		
	You *are* writing.		
	They *are* watching animals.		
	Yesterday my Mom and Dad *were* working.		
	At six o' clock yesterday, we *were* eating dinner.		

Figure 2–1. continues

Morpheme	Example	Correct	Incorrect
Copula (*is, was, are, were*)	This *is* a tiny car.		
	That *is* a big book.		
	My teacher *was* nice to me yesterday.		
	Yesterday, my Mom *was* happy.		
	My friends *are* nice.		
	These trees *are* tall.		
	After the school yesterday, we *were* all hungry.		
	Animals *were* free when they were in the jungle.		

Summary of child's morphologic skills:

_____

_____

_____

Figure 2–1. continued

After calculating MLU, we can engage in play therapy by setting up the therapy room with various objects, toys and books. We can simply be good models and follow the child's lead (see later discussion of Facilitative Play and the Hanen approach). Some clinicians I have known over the years believe that the presence of an adult in the room with one-on-one attention to the child, labeling toys and *consistently* describing/narrating what is going on in the child's play contributes substantially to the child's language. Because we don't want to be known as professionals "who just play with children," we will provide ongoing measurements of growth in MLU over the course of play therapy. As soon as possible, it is imperative to begin requiring more from the child verbally. One of the most effective ways of doing this is to omit one or two of the last words in a particular phrase you have used repeatedly in a play scenario. For instance, if you've been playing "dinner time" and you've been modeling "I want more potatoes," begin to withhold the last word or two "I want more _____," and then "I want _____ _____" allowing the child to fill in more and more of the words. Another effective way to help promote a child's verbalizations is to have him or her fill in more of the words at the end of phrases or sentences that she or he has heard you reading a few times. For instance, when reading *Going on a Bear Hunt* (Rosen, 1989), you read the repetitive phrases: "we can't go over it, we can't go under it . . . we've gotta go through it" a number of times throughout the book. Then start telling the child "I need your help, you need to tell me what this part says" (pointing to the repetitive phrases). You start with "Oh No, Grass. Long, Wavy Grass. We can't go over it. We can't go under it. We've gotta go _____ _____." Soon omit more words: "Oh no, a river. A deep cold river. We can't go over it. We can't go under it. We've _____ _____ _____ _____." I have found that adding gestures to going over and under and through encourage a child to imitate both the gestures and the words.

In addition to describing what's going on during the play, we are guided by the work of early researchers, namely, Roger Brown (1973) and Laura Lee (1974), in the kinds of words typically developing children tend to use as they expand their mean length of utterances. Lee's work is summarized in the next section.

Words to Emphasize When the Child's MLU Is 1.5–2

Indefinite Pronouns or Noun Modifiers: it, this, that

Personal Pronouns: I, me, my, mine, you, your(s)

Main Verbs: Uninflected verbs: I see you; copula: is (He is happy) or 's: (It's red); Auxillary is + verb + ing
(He is running)

Negatives: it, this, that + copula or auxiliary is, 's, + not: It's not mine; This is not a dog; That is not moving

Interrogative Reversals: reversal of copula: Isn't it red? Were they there?

Words to Emphasize When the Child's MLU Is 2–2.5

Indefinite Pronouns or Noun Modifiers: no, some, more, all, lot(s) one(s) two, other(s), another, something, somebody, someone

Personal Pronouns: third person: he, him, his, she, her, hers

Plurals: we, us, our(s), they, them, their, these, those

Main Verbs: -s and –ed: plays, played

Irregular Past: ate, saw

Copula: is (My cat is black) am, are, was, were

Auxiliary: is (He is playing), am, are, was, were

Secondary Verbs: Infinitives: I wanna see; I'm gonna see; I gotta see; Lemme see; Let's play

Noncomplementing Infinitives: I stopped to play; I'm afraid to look; It's hard to do that

WH-Questions: who, what, what + noun (Who am I? What is he eating? What book are you reading? where, how many, how much, what . . . do, what . . . for? Where did it go? How much do you want? What is he doing? What is a hammer for?

Conjunctions: and

Words to Emphasize When the Child's MLU Is 2.5–3.0

Indefinite Pronouns or Noun Modifiers: nothing, nobody, none, no one

Main Verbs: can, will, may + verb, you may go

Obligatory do + verb: don't go

Emphatic do + verb: I do see

Secondary Verbs: participle, present or past: I see a boy running. I found the toy broken

Negatives: can't, don't

Interrogative Reversals: reversal of auxiliary be: Is he throwing? Isn't he throwing? Was he throwing? Wasn't he throwing?

Words to Emphasize When the Child's MLU Is 3.0–3.5

Personal Pronouns: Reflexives: myself, yourself, himself, herself, itself, themselves

Secondary Verbs: early infinitival complements with differing subjects in kernels: I want you to jump. Let him run. Later infinitival complements: I had to run. I told him to go. I tried to run. He ought to run.

Obligatory Deletions: Make it go. I'd better go.

Infinitive with Wh-Word: I know what to get. I know how do do it.

Negatives: isn't, won't

Conjunctions: but, so, and so, so that, or, if

Wh-Quesions: when, how, how + adjective: When shall I run? How do you do it? How green is it?

Words to Emphasize When the Child's MLU Is 3.5–4

Personal Pronouns: wh-pronouns: who, which, whose, whom, what, that, how many, how much, I know who came. That's what I said

Wh-word + Infinitive: I know what to do; I know who(m) to take

Main Verbs: could, would, should, might + verb

    Obligatory does, did + verb

    Emphatic does, did + verb

Conjunctions: because

Interrogative Reversals:

    Obligatory: do, does, did: Do they run? Does it bite/ Didn't it hurt?

    Reversal of modal: Can you play? Won't it hurt? Shall I sit down?

    Tag question: It's fun isn't it? It isn't fun, is it?

Words to Emphasize When the Child's MLU Is 4–4.5

Indefinite Pronouns or Noun Modifiers:

    Any, anything, anybody, anyone

    Every, everything, everybody, everyone

    Both, few, many, each, several, most, least, much, next, first, last, second.

Personal Pronouns: his own, one, oneself, whichever, whoever, whatever. Take whatever you like.

Main Verbs: passive with get, any tense; passive with be, any tense

    Must, shall + verb: must run

    Have + verb + en: I've eaten

    Have got: I've got it

Secondary Verbs: passive infinitival complement:

    With get: I have to get dressed; I don't want to get hurt

    With be: I want to be pulled; It's going to be locked

Negatives:

    Uncontracted negatives: I can not go; he has not gone

Pronoun-auxiliary or pronoun-copula contraction: I'm not coming here; He's not here

Auxiliary-negative or copula-negative contractions: He wasn't going; he hasn't been seen; it couldn't be mine; they aren't big; he didn't

Wh-Questions: why, what if, how come, how about + gerund: Why are you crying: What if I won't do it? How come he is crying? How about coming with me?

Words to Emphasize When the Child's MLU Is 4.5–5

Main Verbs:

Have/had been + verb + ing

Modal + have + verb + en: may have eaten

Modal + be + verb + ing: could be playing

Other auxiliary combinations: should have been sleeping

Secondary Verbs:

Gerund: swinging (add ing) is fun; I like fishing; he started laughing

Conjunctions:

Where, when, how, while, whether (or not) til, until, unless, since, before, after, for, as, as + adjective + as, as if, like, that, than I know where you are; don't go till I say

Obligatory deletions: I run faster than you (run); I'm as big as a man (is big); It looks like a dog (looks)

Elliptical deletions: That's why (I took it); I know how (I can do it)

Wh-words + infinitive: I know how to do it

Interrogative Reversals:

Reversal of auxiliary: have: Has he seen you?

Reversal with two or there auxiliaries: Has he been eating? Couldn't he have waited? Could he have been crying: Wouldn't he have been going

Wh-Questions: whose, which, which + noun: Whose car is that? Which book do you want?

Figure 2–1 on page 22 provides an assessment protocol for grammatic morphemes.

What Are Some Techniques to Use in Early Phases of Child Language Therapy?

A multitude of materials exist on the topic of how to do child language therapy. Techniques generally vary from the adult following the child's lead to the adult modeling and expanding what the child is saying, to a very directive role in which the adult asks the child to "say this." I will briefly introduce some of the ideas here from information on *facilitative play* and the *Hanen approach*.

I had the wonderful opportunity during my tenure at California State University, Sacramento, to work with Dr. Robert Hubbell. We supervised together as well as team-taught a graduate level language disorders class. Dr. Hubbell proposed using *facilitative play* as a technique for encouraging maximal talking in children. Facilitative play promotes low structured modeling of language structures and conversational strategies by adults, collecting language samples, and "outwitting some resistant children." The following information is abstracted from a handout Dr. Hubbell used in his teachings at California State University, Sacramento. According to Hubbell (1996), facilitate play is based on two key factors that encourage maximal talking in children:

1. **Topic of immediate interest to the child:** meaning whatever the child is attending to at the moment, regardless of any favorite topics we believe a child to have.
2. **Power relations between child and adult de-emphasize the adult's image as power figure and authority.** As much as possible, adult and child are "equals," rather than the child being one-down and the adult one-up.

Although Hubbell proposed that ultimately, facilitative play becomes an attitude toward children and how to approach them rather than a set of techniques, he offered the following five suggestions to consider while engaging in facilitative play techniques.

1. **Appealing activities.** Offer a variety of high-interest activities to the child. Have different activities available: not three picture games, but some pictures, some blocks, a play house, a kitchen area, and so forth. Strive for activities that children just "naturally" like to do.
2. **Follow the child's lead.** Encourage the child to select the activities, and go along with the child in how those activities are pursued. When the child changes, you change, and so on.
3. **Avoid directing the child.** Resist the temptation to elicit responses, demonstrate how things work, suggest activities, and so forth. On the other hand, keep some basic limits. Children shouldn't hit, grind clay into the carpet, or engage in other destructive activities.
4. **Talk about what the child is doing.** You may narrate, converse, or make your talk part of the play. Ideally, the clinician talks less than the child does. In suggestion 3 above, avoid frequent questions and commands, and veiled directives of one sort or another.
5. **Use language of appropriate level for the child.** The goal of facilitative play is not to teach specific grammatical structures, but it is helpful to use language that is at the child's level.

The *Hanen* approach for early intervention is particularly useful when working with toddlers and preschool children. As McCauley and Fey (2006) pointed out, the goal of the Hanen approach is to increase parents' use of general interaction strategies to facilitate children's communication. "This intervention program has been used effectively with late-talking toddlers and preschool-age children with developmental delays (e.g., Down syndrome)" (Girolametto & Weitzman, 2006, p. 77). The reader of this resource is encouraged to read the book by Pepper and Weitzman (2004) among many other resources and publications provided through the Hanen Centre as well as attend one the Hanen training workshops. See http://www.hanen.org

A primary strength of the Hanen program is the training of speech-language pathologists in Hanen techniques to train parents to do the same with their children. Parents are first encouraged to identify which of the following communicators their child might be.

Discoverer: reacts to how he or she feels and what is happening in his or her immediate surroundings but not communicating with specific purpose in mind.

Communicator: sends specific messages without use of words.

First Word Users: uses single words, signs, or pictures.

Combiners: combine words into two- to three-word utterances.

Among the vast number of suggestions provided in the workshops and in the book by Pepper and Weitzman (2004) are the following few. Parents and SLPs are encouraged to OWL: *observe* the child; *wait* for the child to react by stop talking, leaning forward, and looking at the child expectantly; and *listen* by paying close attention to what the child is doing or saying. The Hanen manual offers suggestions as to how to encourage the child to talk, to add to what is being said, and so forth through the use of books and music. An invaluable source!

Techniques to Add Into Facilitative Play and Hanen

More directive approaches are described in a number of sources on child language therapy. In these approaches, the adult is more directive than in the approaches described above through modeling or expanding what he or she wants the child to say. See Chapter 5 in this resource for more "unnatural" techniques known as "hybrid" and "clinician directed" approaches to child language intervention.

An approach that might be described as somewhere between facilitative play and Hanen approaches, or one that offers techniques to incorporate into these two techniques, is known as a "child-centered (CC) approach." In her description of this approach, Paul (2007) reminded us that "you can lead a horse to water, but you can't make it drink" (p. 76). This is the potential problem when using more clinician-directed (CD) approaches. As Paul explained, "some children simply refuse to engage in CD activities . . . these 'hard-to-treat' children rebuff any attempt to get them to say what the clinician tells them to say, no matter how tempting the reinforcement" (p. 76). In explaining the benefits of CC therapy approach, Paul maintained that, as in the Hanen approach, we must wait. "The key to this approach is to respond to the client. To do this, we have to wait for the client to do something. Ideally, that something will be to talk" (p. 77). If the child talks, the CC approach offers some specific verbal techniques to facilitate more talking. Paul summarized these techniques as follows:

> **Self-Talk:** involves the clinician describing his or her own actions as he or she engages in parallel play with the child. As with all parallel play, the adult does what the child does and comments from a "first person" standpoint. For example, you may be copying what a child is doing in drawing the picture of a face, commenting: "I'm drawing. I drew a mouth, and a nose, and eyes." "Self-talk provides a clear and simple match between actions and words" (Paul, 2007, p. 77).

> **Parallel Talk:** like self-talk, parallel talk supplies ongoing commentary for what is happening in your play. Rather than using first person "I" statements, the clinician uses third person comments such as "You are drawing. You drew a mouth, and a nose and eyes."

> **Imitation:** involves the adult imitating the child. Paul cited research showing that, when an adult imitates verbalizations of a typically developing child, there is a "substantial probability that the child will imitate the imitation" (p. 77).

> **Expansion:** when expanding a child's utterance, the adult repeats what the child has said and models correct grammatical markers and semantic details. When a child says something like "mommy car," we're not always sure as to the semantic relations underlying the form of the comment. If the child has put a play mommy into a car, the adult can expand with "Mommy is in her car." If the child shows you a picture of his or her mommy next to her car and says

"mommy car," we can expand the utterance with "right, that is mommy's car."

Extensions: add to what the child has just said. As Paul noted, extensions "are comments that add some semantic information to a remark made by the child" (p. 78). With the child's comment about "mommy car," the adult can add, "that's mommy's red car," or "mommy parked her car by your house."

Buildups and Breakdowns: involve expanding what a child has said followed by breaking the utterance back down into discrete parts. In a play situation where play has involved an airplane and the child has commented "airplane fly," the adult can build this up with "yes, the airplane is flying high in the sky." The adult then breaks the utterance back down into "the airplane is flying high," the airplane is flying," "airplane fly."

Recast Sentences: provide the child with a different type or more elaborated sentence than the child produced. Using the "airplane" example above, if the child comments "airplane fly," the adult can recast the comment into a negative statement: "The airplane did not fly there," or a question: "Did the airplane fly?" or a past tense "The airplane flew home."

Potpourri

Before leaving this chapter, I'd like to mention that my own "recipe" for therapy with young children is to combine facilitative techniques and gradually to interject more directive child-centered techniques. I may begin and return to following the child's lead, then interject parallel talk, expansion, and so forth. I am also a strong proponent of Language is the Key as described by Cole, Maddox, and Lim. (2006). In this approach, picture books are used to provide a tool for interaction between child and adult in both emergent and literacy skills. After working with children in promoting early verbalizations through facilitative play and/or Hanen approaches, when the child begins to show some boredom with play activities and begins to show more interest in books, I introduce books. According to Cole et al., when adults look at books with children during play, some techniques include:

1. making comments about the child's interests,
2. asking questions related to the child's interests, and
3. responding to child utterances by adding a little more information (p. 149).

I also think it is appropriate to let children know that it is not okay to shrug their shoulders or ignore the adult talking with them. I frequently say to children, "we use words here, you need to use your words." I have a speech pathologist friend who believes that, if children *could* say their words, they would. I believe that if some children had the words in their repertoire they might try them out if encouraged to do so. I also believe that children with language issues learn very early to stop taking risks (see Chapter 5 regarding learned helplessness and cognitive rigidity). How many times does it take for other children and adults in their environment saying "Huh?" "What did you say?" to discourage even the bravest child with limited verbal abilities from trying to talk? I simply get "pushy" from time to time with a reluctant communicator who, in my mind, needs to be introduced or reminded how the communication game is played.

The purpose of this chapter was to demonstrate how to incorporate many of the rich sources available on children's play into a resource linking the strands of language and literacy. To that end, the following questions were addressed:

■ How does children's play develop?
■ What do children talk about?
■ What are various types of children's play?
■ What kind of concepts do young children acquire?
■ What are specific word types and words to emphasize at various MLUs?
■ What are some techniques to use in early phases of child language therapy?

It is now time to move to link to the next language-literacy strand, namely, listening skills. Although the notion of auditory processing disorders will be discussed briefly, the intent of Chapter 3 is to answer questions that students and seasoned practitioners continually ask as to which listening skills are critical to scaffolding/supporting children's developing language systems.

Remember: your client may need to have *play* targeted as the first strand to include in his or her language therapy *or* she or he may need to revisit this strand while working on later strands.

Chapter 3

Listening Skills

Background

The listening skills strand is critical for a child's developing oral-written language system. Like so many areas in child language, a discussion of listening skills brings with it a need for defining terms. In this area, questions arise as to whether we are referring to central auditory processing, to auditory processing, or as Bellis (2001) cleverly said: or is it "George?" For purposes of this resource, the term auditory processing will be used. Across the country, the term "auditory processing problem" is met with a great deal of confusion—to the point that some school district personnel would simply like the term to "go away." What's more, many descriptions of "auditory processing problems" overlap with descriptions of children diagnosed with various language disorders.

To add to the confusion, children with language disorders are described by different terms such as "specific language disorder," "garden variety language disability," or "language learning disabled." Furthermore, terms used to describe conditions change over time. As Johnston (2006) reflected: "The first conference on a condition known as 'childhood aphasia' was held at Stanford University in 1960. Forty-five years later, the name has changed to 'specific language impairment' (SLI), but the nature of the condition remains a puzzle. Language is, after all, a product of the mind. If it doesn't develop on the predicted course, some mental function must be implicated" (p. 31).

There seems to be overlapping, nonexclusive characteristics in children with auditory processing and language processing problems and included in many of their descriptions is a deficit in *listening skills*. Are their language problems the result of fundamental listening skills deficits? Or do the receptive/expressive language problems these children present with negatively impact their listening skills? Do we have a chicken-egg scenario here? Or do we have something similar to the fable of the Six Blind Men and the Elephant where each of the blind men touched a different part of the elephant describing the elephant as the specific part touched by each blind man? How many times have we attended college lectures, sessions at professional meetings, or finished reading a journal article describing something about children with auditory processing problems and commented to ourselves or a colleague: "Boy, that sounds just like my language-learning disabled client or my client with specific language impairment."

(Central) Auditory Processing Disorder

The California Speech-Language-Hearing Association (CSHA) Position Paper on Auditory Processing Disorder (2002) included the following description of auditory skills: "Auditory processing is not a singular skill, but rather an integration of skills that are basic to the listening and communication process. The boundaries of each are not well defined, resulting in overlap and are, essentially, inseparable" (p. 5). Richard (2007) explained that "part of the dilemma is due to confounding terminology used to describe the disorder, for example, auditory processing, central auditory processing, language processing, sensory processing, and speech perception" (p. 161). To help delineate these terms, Richard explained that, to differentiate auditory processing from language processing is "to acknowledge the acoustic, phonemic, and linguistic roles, both neurologically and behaviorally" (p. 166). A synopsis of her description follows:

- ■ The **peripheral auditory system** is active in auditory processing, which involves reception and transfer of an acoustic signal. The auditory/acoustic processing portion of Richard's model involves the audiologist in two ways:
  1. The peripheral auditory system involves testing of puretone thresholds and tympanometry.

2. The central auditory system involves testing of electro-physiologic aspects; pitch patterns, dichotic digits, and figure-ground.

■ The **central auditory system** is active when the listener discriminates the acoustic signal as being environmental or linguistically encoded within the existing sound system of his or her specific language. Critical here is the listener's knowledge of his or her spoken language's phonetic code allowing him or her to "discriminate and analyze the signal's component parts" (p. 166). In this step, the acoustic/auditory processing task evolves into a phonological processing task, that is, phonemic processing. The phonemic processing portion of Richard's model involves either the audiologist or speech pathologist assessing phoneme discrimination; sound blending; and auditory segmentation.

■ **Language/linguistic processing** now becomes involved in applying the linguistic code to allow the listener to interpret or extrapolate the message. "The individual must transition into language knowledge to comprehend or understand the intention of the speaker" (p. 166). The linguistic processing portion of Richard's model involves the speech pathologist assessing concepts, antonyms, idioms, nonliteral language, and problem solving.

In underscoring the confusion that can result from the above terms, Richard offered the following:

Audiologists typically include assessment tasks that evaluate sound discrimination of phonological segments. The stimuli can include both nonsense and meaningful syllables or words. This portion of the continuum is often the highest level of audiologic assessment, or central auditory processing evaluations. If an individual encounters difficulty at this level, the audiologist will diagnose a *central auditory processing disorder*. However, assessment by a speech-language pathologist should begin in this same portion of the continuum. Evaluation of phonemic awareness can include the same types of tasks as those administered by audiologists, utilizing both nonsense and meaningful stimuli. The speech-language pathologist will diagnose a *language processing or phonological awareness disorder*. Consequently, the exact same deficit can result in three different diagnoses, depending on who first conducts the evaluation. (p. 168)

Johnston (2006) provided a succinct synopsis of the audio-logic/language view of what is going on in this arena. The *audiologic view* represents a narrow, bottom-up view in which "something is adversely affecting the processing or interpretation of the information" (citing National Institutes of Health, 2004, p. 83). This approach emphasizes the processes underlying language rather than higher order language, cognitive, or related factors. Those working from the audiologic view believe that:

1. The mental events involved in the processing of acoustic information are *best* viewed as auditory,
2. CAPD may coexist with other conditions but is *importantly* distinct from them, and
3. The academic, language, and attentional problems seen in many children are actually a manifestation, or result of, CAPD (Johnston, p. 84).

The *language view*, ascribed to primarily by speech-language pathologists, supports a more top-down processing approach emphasizing "learning and communication problems seen in many school-age children are a source, rather than a consequence, of auditory difficulties" (Johnston, p. 85). Citing research on children with specific language impairment, Johnston concluded that the presumed central auditory difficulties in this case "actually reflected poor representation of the speech sound system, and thus that the perceptual deficits had more to do with language than with audition" (p. 85). Finally, the following recommendations were included in the CSHA (2002) position paper:

The audiologic view suggests emphasizing listening skills from a bottom-up approach spending more time on discrete sounds and sound segmentation vs. the language approach emphasizing listening skills as well as clarifying the child's ability to think about the more meaningful aspects of the words in the speech stream. Most professionals in the field feel a *combination* of a "top-down, bottom-up" approach to the treatment of APD is more effective than a singular approach. That is, a combination of interventions that facilitate higher-order ("top-down") linguistic and cognitive skills such as metacognitive strategies or vocabulary development, with the remediation of the underlying auditory deficits ("bottom-up") is the most advantageous approach (ASHA Conference, 2005).

Although many children with APD require therapy for receptive language deficits, it should be recognized that the two interventions do overlap in some areas. However, receptive language development is not a replacement for APD therapy, although it may be necessary to address both areas. (pp. 26–27)

In their technical report, the American Speech-Language-Hearing Association (ASHA, 2005) explained that the term "central" should be placed within parentheses because not everyone includes the term. Thus, (central) auditory processing ([C]AP) "refers to the efficiency and effectiveness by which the central nervous system (CNS) utilizes auditory information. Narrowly defined, (C)AP refers to the perceptual processing of auditory information in the CNS and the neurobiologic activity that underlies that processing and gives rise to electrophysiological auditory potentials" (p. 2). As Luker (2007) pointed out, the ASHA report goes on to say "that APD can lead to problems in higher order or levels of processing involving language, communication, and learning as well as . . . can coexist with other disorders such as AD/HD, language impairment, and learning disabilities" (p. 14).

An interesting alternative view is presented by those who support an information-processing view of listening skills. Benson (1994) suggested that thinking "represents the activities of a number of diverse, precisely interrelated nervous system functions that process thought contents" (p. 5). Cognition, which is one step in the process of thinking, "is the process by which information is manipulated in the brain" (p. 5). Thought processing "demands interrelationships" among nine functional systems: sensory (visual, auditory, tactile), motor, basic mental control, emotion/autonomic, memory, visual imagery, language, cognition, and higher mental control (Benson, p. 25). Auditory processing comprises one of the functional systems engaged in ongoing activity during thought processing and is always occurring as the brain recognizes and interprets heard sounds. Stated differently, auditory processing is ongoing and nonintentional. Johnston (2006) summarized some of the beliefs of proponents of an information-processing view:

■ Instead of viewing language impairment as a specific disorder, an information-processing view considers this condition as a consequence of deficits in general information processing mechanisms.

■ For children with SLI, language may present the most obvious learning challenges, but attention and memory difficulties extend into nonverbal areas as well.

■ In contrast to the audiologists who define (C)APD as a deficit that "is not due to higher-order language, cognitive or related factors" (citing ASHA, 2005, p. 2), "proponents of an information processing alternative argue that the difficulties with auditory processing are exactly a direct consequence of those higher order factors."

■ In an information processing alternative, the auditory nature of the stimuli does not define the problem.

■ "Instead, auditory processing difficulties are just one manifestation of a broader cognitive processing deficiency which is likely to cause other learning and performance deficits as well" (Johnston, p. 86).

Many researchers, authors, and practitioners discuss the overlapping of symptomatology among auditory processing and language processing disorders. In their discussion of "Comorbidity of APD with Other 'Look-Alikes,'" Hamaguchi and Tazeau (2007) reminded, us as medical professionals often say, "When you hear hoof-beats, you can't just think of horses" (p. 50). Although these authors discussed the comorbidity of APD and a number of attentional and linguistic problems, the focus here will remain with the overlap of symptomatology that APD has with specific language impairment (SLI) and language learning disabilities (LLD).

Ross-Swain and Geffner (2009) listed the following behaviors frequently exhibited by children with (C)APD:

■ Poor listening skills
■ Difficulty learning through the auditory modality
■ Difficulty following auditory instructions
■ Short auditory memory span
■ Difficulty understanding in the presence of background noise
■ Frequently saying "huh?" and "what?"
■ Poor auditory memory for commands and sequences
■ Tend to recall the last part of a sequence and forget what is said soon after
■ Tend to give slow or delayed responses to verbal stimuli
■ Misunderstand what is said or "mishear"

- Difficulty understanding speech that has been muffled or distorted
- Poor attention and focusing
- Easily distracted primarily by noise
- Poor speech recognition in noise
- They may have better-than-normal hearing, or hypersensitivity
- Auditory integration deficits for sound blending and auditory closure, phonological awareness, and "phonic" skills (p. 2).

In their 2008 presentation, Ross-Swain and Geffner included additional descriptions of receptive-expressive and pragmatic language problems frequently demonstrated by children with (C)APD:

- They present with receptive language problems due to: limited auditory memory; reauditorization and temporal sequencing deficits; linguistic processing deficits, with poor interpretation of ambiguous sentences, idioms, puns, jokes, analogies; increased latency in responding.
- They present with expressive language problems including: paraphasic errors; word finding difficulty; word substitution errors; delay in onset of expressive language; difficulty expressing feelings; poor use of referents; sequencing difficulties; difficulties with nonliteral meanings; overshooting main idea; poor organization of thought; and produce less information and organized narratives.
- They present with pragmatic problems that include: difficulties in social context; limited exchange of greetings; difficulty expressing intent; limitations in inquiring; limitations in requesting information; difficulty initiating/terminating conversation; difficulty maintaining topic; and difficulty in problem solving and planning.

Specific Language Impairment

Specific language impairment (SLI) is a developmental language disorder in the absence of other cognitive, known neurologic, sensorimotor, or social emotional deficits (Watkins & Kadem 1994). The impairment is specific, that is, limited, to language. Children who develop SLI may develop language slower than their typically developing peers and are often referred to as "late bloomers," but usually are not diagnosed until around 4 years of age. Compared to their typically developing peers, children with SLI make slow progress in developing language skills. Some researchers attribute the source of their difficulty to a deficit in processing brief rapidly changing auditory information and/or remembering the temporal order of the auditory information (Tallal, Stark, & Mellits, 1985). Leonard, Eyer, Bedore, and Greta (1997) suggested this difficulty with rapidly changing auditory information may lead to problems perceiving grammatical forms, such as "the" and "is," as these are generally brief in duration. A second hypothesis as to the SLI child's difficulty with morphology stems from difficulty or delays in acquiring a specific underlying linguistic mechanism that facilitates acquiring rules, for instance, that verbs must be marked for tense and number ("the dog barks" not "bark"). Yet a third hypothesis was offered by Baddeley, Gathercole, and Papagno (1998) suggesting the difficulties seen in SLI result from poor short-term memory for verbal material as opposed to nonverbal or environmental sounds. Hegde and Pomaville (2008) included the following characteristics in their description of children with SLI:

Errors in speech production: Omission of speech sounds such as /t/, /d/, /s/, or /z/ will not be able to mark regular past tense t or d (*walked* or *begged*), the third person singular present tense (e.g., *walks*), the possessive morpheme (e.g., *Mommy's*), and regular plural words (e.g., *bats* or *bags*).

Semantic problems: According to these authors "difficulty learning words and their meanings is an early sign of SLI. Children with SLI are slow to acquire their first few words and fail to show the typical explosive increase in the acquisition of new words between the ages of 18 and 24 months." They may also overextend (e.g., calling all adults "Daddy") and underextend (e.g., only the family dog is called "dog") the use of words beyond the age of 3 years. (p. 217)

Delayed word combinations: Children with SLI may be slower in combining two words.

Naming errors: School-age children with SLI demonstrate difficulty naming pictured objects.

Difficulty with abstract and figurative language: As children with SLI grow older and into adolescence, they reveal problems with more abstract language forms such as proverbs, idioms, similes, and other figurative language.

Significant morphologic problems: Problems producing morphologic features of language is a diagnostic feature of SLI.

Limited syntactic structure and variety: simpler sentence forms; lack of syntactic variety; absence of complex, compound, embedded, and passive sentence forms; and difficulty in transforming one type of sentence (e.g., active declarative) to another form (e.g., a question) all characterize the language skills of children with SLI.

Controversial pragmatic language problems: possibly, topic initiation and maintenance, turn-taking skills, and conversational repair strategies will be less impaired than joint attention, detailed and sophisticated narration of stories or personal experiences, group interactions and discussions, and discussion of advanced academic topics. (pp. 217–218)

Language Learning Disabilities

Children with *language learning disabilities* (LLD) have normal cognitive abilities and therefore are not considered to be "slow learners." These are children who are not considered as impaired in language as in the case of developmental aphasia or developmental language disorders. Some may use LLD synonymously with SLI. Children with LLD have a selective language impairment and do not learn in a typical way when language is involved. Because they present with slower speech and language developmental milestones, their problems appear in preschool when they are identified and usually receive speech and language services. Because they benefit from early language intervention, they eventually do develop these early language skills. They tend to be discharged from therapy yet have lingering problems with language as the academics challenge them (Prifitera, Saktofske, & Weiss, 2004). Paul (2001) described the following characteristics of students with LLD.

Phonological Characteristics

About 25% of children with LLD have delayed speech development at school age, although most are intelligible. They often have difficulty with complex phonological production, that is, producing phonologically complex, multisyllabic words (aluminum) or phrases (I pledge allegiance to the flag). Children with slow language development during preschool period may be at risk for LLD.

Students with LLD tend to have difficulty with short-term memory problems involving verbal material but not nonverbal environmental sounds; difficulty rapidly naming automatized sequences such as days of the week; difficulty repeating nonwords, and may have word-retrieval problems. Although these difficulties may not seem phonologically based, "researchers believe that the source . . . is in establishing and retrieving accurate phonological representations (or segmenting the words into sounds, then storing sound-by-sound auditory images and retrieving these images as a template for production) of verbal material" (Paul, 2007, p. 436). Baddeley et al. (1998) described the problem with verbal short-term memory as a diminished ability of the articulatory/phonological loop to function efficiently enough to allow the child (in this case) to mentally replay the exact replica of what he or she heard. The phonologic loop supports the learning of new vocabulary words and it may "mediate the acquisition of syntactic knowledge" (p. 9). These authors explained that one of the ways typically developing children rapidly learn syntactic rules is through "learning a storehouse of multiword language patterns that are used to abstract rules that govern connected language" (p. 9). If a weakened, and thereby less efficient, phonologic loop negatively impacts a child's ability to store these multiword language patterns, he or she has less material from which to abstract the syntactic rules governing language. Baddeley et al. also cited Speidel's (1993) work indicating that multiword utterances must be held in a phonologic working memory. In order for raw utterances or constructions to be learned accurately and fast depends on how accurately their initially held phonologic representations are. Once again, the inference is on the integrity of the phonologic buffer to "replay" and store words and syntactic constructions heard to be able to "move" them to long-term memory.

Paul (2007) cited others (e.g., Catts & Kamhi, 2005) who are among those who believe "that dyslexia may be a very specific disorder of phonological processing" (p. 435). The metalinguistic activity of breaking the speech stream into words, syllables, and phonemes, known as phonological awareness, has been found to be critical to successfully learning to read an alphabetic language and frequently weakened in students with developmental dyslexia (see Chapter 5). With regard to more general reading, Paul cited Snowling, Bishop, and Stothard (2000) who reported "reading outcomes are poorest for children with the most severe phonological disorders" (p. 435).

Syntactic Characteristics

Students with LLD may experience difficulty comprehending complex syntax, particularly those with relative clauses, passive voice, or negation. Whereas typically developing children move to full comprehension of complex syntax by 7 to 8 years, children with LLD continue to rely on comprehension strategies for passive sentences and those with relative and adverbial clauses. For instance, "Students with LLD persist in misinterpreting sentences such as 'before you brush your teeth, put away your towel,' in which the order of clauses ('brush teeth,' 'put away towel') is opposite of the intended order of events (first put away towel, then brush teeth)" (Paul, 2007, pp. 436–437). Although children with LLD do not make large numbers of syntactic errors in spontaneous speech, they have a tendency to produce "simple" or "immature" sentences with fewer complex sentences, using fewer multiple modifiers, prepositional phrases, relative clauses, and verb phrases (p. 437). Although their sentences may "actually be longer than those of peers, because they use fewer complex forms to condense their expression (Paul, citing Kuder, 1997), they tend to "talk around the issue" rather than specifically defining a problem or describing something succinctly and difficulty "hooking" the referent (the person or thing being talked about) with their corresponding pronouns. I am forever asking my LLD students to tell me who they are talking about, or who said what to whom. Scott (2004) found that morphological problems account for two-thirds of the syntactic errors in students with LLD.

Semantic Characteristics

Students with LLD tend to have smaller vocabularies, restricted to high-frequency, short words. Their vocabulary problems result, in part, from reading problems. They have restricted word meanings, and poor associations among words and categorization of words into semantic classes. They typically have problems with multiple-meaning words and may rely on nonspecific terms (thing, stuff). They have difficulty with relational and abstract words and may have word-retrieval problems with many instances of substitution and circumlocution in their spontaneous speech. They also may have difficulty understanding complex oral directions, difficulty understanding and using figurative language, and problems integrating meaning across sentences (Paul 2007, p. 437).

Pragmatic Characteristics

Students with LLD typically present with limited verbal output and fluency and their speech can be characterized by dysfluencies caused by many false starts. Their verbal output tends to be less polite, persuasive, assertive, clear, and complete, and is less sensitive to listeners' needs. They frequently give incomplete or inaccurate descriptions and they experience difficulty clarifying miscommunications and requesting clarification. They are likely to ignore communicative bids of others, and have poor topic maintenance (Paul, 2007, pp. 437–438).

This overview of auditory and language processing problems was included to illustrate some of the confusion that exists between and among terms. The purpose of this chapter is not to argue that one problem exists while the other does not. Certainly, there can be agreement that children with auditory processing problems and those with language processing problems share some listening skill problems needing remediation. To assess or work only on listening skills to the exclusion of language skills or assessing and working on language skills to the exclusion of listening skills in children with listening and language processing problems is shortsighted.

Notes on Assessment

The diagnosis of auditory processing disorders is the role of the audiologist (ASHA, 2005). According to this report, "SLPs have a unique role in delineating cognitive-communicative and language-related factors that may be associated with (C)APD in some individuals, and in the differential diagnosis of language processing disorders from (C)APD" (p. 6). The California Language Speech and Hearing Association (2002) proposed the following in attempting to differentiate auditory processing disorders from language processing disorders.

> An auditory processing disorder and a language disorder are not synonymous terms. Not all APDs lead to language disorders and not all language disorders are due to APDs. There are many reasons a child has difficulty with processing language aside from an auditory processing disorder. Language comprehension tests should not be used to diagnose an auditory processing disorder, although behaviors and response patterns observed may indicate the need for further testing in the area of auditory processing. Pure language processing (comprehension) tests only require the child to point to a picture or follow a verbal direction. As soon as a verbal response is required, the answer is affected by the child's expressive language and is then measuring two components, and great care must be taken when interpreting test results to determine if the presence of an expressive language disorder is present.
>
> An *auditory processing* assessment focuses on evaluating how the child is receiving speech sound(s), depending upon the auditory context, acoustic features of the speech signal, and environment. It seeks to determine if the auditory speech signal is reaching the child's language centers intact, in the same way other people perceive it. For example, if a child exhibits a significant left-ear weakness on auditory testing, it indicates a discrepancy that is typical for a child with APD and probably not the result of a language processing problem.
>
> A *language processing* assessment focuses on how the child processes the verbal information *after* it has been delivered by the auditory system. It focuses on evaluating if the child comprehends specific word meanings and sentence types such as those used in following directions, passive voice, categorization, idioms, prepositions, "wh" questions, etc. (p. 14)

In a unique coverage of the SLP's role in assessment of APD, Ross-Swain (2007) offered a number of suggestions. She cautioned "keep in mind that the information that the speech-language pathologist is providing is not a diagnosis but rather a reporting of auditory processing skill weaknesses that impact language, cognition, and memory" (p. 147). Included among tests suggested by Geffner and Ross-Swain (2008) are the following.

Tests for Assessing Skills of Auditory Perception and Discrimination

1. The Goldman-Fristoe-Woodcock Test of Auditory Discrimination, Quiet Subtest
2. The Lindamood Auditory Conceptualization Test-Third Edition (LAC-3)
3. The Test of Auditory Processing Skills-Third Edition (TAPS-3)
4. The Test of Language Development-Third Edition (TOLD-3)
5. Wepman's Auditory Discrimination Test

Tests for Assessing Skills of Auditory Memory

1. The Auditory Processing Abilities Test Subtests: 2, 6, and 9
2. The Clinical Evaluation of Language Fundamentals, Fourth Edition (CELF-4) Subtests: Concepts and Following Directions, Number Repetition, and Familiar Sequences
3. The Comprehensive Test of Phonological Processing (CTOPP) Subtest III
4. The Test Language Development-Primary-Third Edition (TOLD-P3) Subtest V
5. The Token Test for Children
6. The Test of Auditory Processing Skills-Third Edition (TAPS-3) Subtests: Number Memory Forward; Number Memory Reversed; Word Memory, and Sentence Memory
7. Wepman's Auditory Memory Battery
8. The Wide Range Assessment of Memory and Learning-Second Edition (WRAML-2)

Tests for Assessing Skills of Phonemic Awareness

1. The Auditory Processing Abilities Test (APAT) Subtest 1
2. The Clinical Evaluation of Language Fundamentals, Fourth Edition (CELF-4) Subtest: Phonological Awareness
3. The Comprehensive Test of Phonological Processing (CTOPP) Subtests 1, 2, 8, 10, 11, and 12
4. The Lindamood Auditory Conceptualization Test-Third Edition (LAC-3)
5. The Phonological Awareness Test

6. The Test of Language Development-Primary-Third Edition (TOLD-P3)
7. The Test of Auditory Processing Skills-Third Edition (TAPS-3) Subtests: Phonological Segmentation and Phonological Blending

Tests for Assessing Skills of Auditory Closure

1. The Comprehensive Assessment of Spoken Language (CASL) Subtest: Meaning from Context
2. Test of Language Competence (TLC) Subtest 3

Tests for Assessing Skills of Auditory Comprehension and Auditory Cohesion

1. The Auditory Processing Abilities Test (APAT) Subtests 7, 8, 10
2. The Clinical Evaluation of Language Fundamentals, Fourth Edition (CELF-4) Subtests: Linguistic Concepts, Sentence Structure, Concepts and Directions and Understanding Spoken Paragraphs
3. The Comprehensive Assessment of Spoken Language (CASL) Subtests: Sentence Comprehension, Paragraph Comprehension, Nonliteral Language Ambiguous Sentences and Inference
4. The Listening Test
5. The Test of Auditory Processing Skills-Third Edition (TAPS 3) Subtests: Auditory Comprehension and Auditory Reasoning
6. The Test for Language Competence (TLC) Subtests 1 and 4
7. The Token Test for Children
8. The Wide Range Assessment of Memory and Learning-Second Edition (WRAML-2) Subtests 1 and 6

Additionally, Ross-Swain (2007) offered suggestions to help SLPs identify how weaknesses in specific auditory processing skills affect children in specific learning processes. These are summarized briefly below:

Effects of auditory discrimination problem: student has difficulty with:

- understanding directions
- following directions, which may appear to be the result of auditory memory problems. "Careful analysis and interpretation of testing can assist in 'sorting out' what

is more likely the actual cause of a child's difficulty with following directions" (Ross-Swain, p. 155)

■ figuring out what was said (e.g., in a receptive language task such as "pick up the _____" and miss the remainder of the direction/instruction
■ getting his or her work completed, working "overtime" listening to what is being said
■ staying tuned in due to resulting fatigue

Effects of auditory memory skills problem: student has difficulty with:

■ following age-appropriate multistep directions
■ comprehending paragraph material presented auditorily
■ holding information in auditory memory resulting in losing information that overloads memory capacity. This may result in the student beginning to focus on new information being delivered that may not be related to what was previously being delivered. As an example, this student is able to hold information A in his or her auditory memory, "lose related information B," and focus on unrelated information C. This causes the student to work "overtime" trying to understand unrelated fragmented bits of information

Effects of auditory processing delays: student has difficulty with:

■ following verbally presented directions
■ comprehending spoken information
■ daydreaming or tuning out
■ teachers/parents often complain "If he would pay attention he could listen better"

Effects of auditory processing/phonemic awareness skills: Ross-Swain summarized Gillet's (1993) work high-lighting the resulting problems the student with auditory processing problems may have with reading and spelling.

■ Difficulty hearing similarities in initial and final sounds in words
■ Difficulty hearing adjacent sounds in consonant blends

- Difficulty discriminating short vowel sounds
- Difficulty rhyming
- Difficulty breaking words into syllables or individual sounds
- Difficulty retaining each of the sounds or syllables
- Difficulty blending sounds together as a whole, even though the individual sounds are known
- Difficulty remembering the sound of a letter or how to say a word, even though the meaning may be known
- Difficulty imprecisely relating the auditory symbol with the visual symbol
- May substitute words when reading aloud and/or
- May distort the pronunciation of multisyllabic words due to difficulty in sequencing sounds (pp. 154–155).

In an attempt to understand problems in and teaching techniques to enhance listening problems, Ferre (2000), Bellis (2001), and Bellis (2003) identified three primary subtypes of auditory processing problems. They have been included here because SLPs often receive reports by audiologists using terminology included in the following subtypes. They have been included here under subtype headings for the practitioner who is working with a client/student following an audiologist's evaluation and diagnosis of an auditory processing disorder, and for the practitioner who is working with a client/student with language problems, which may result in listening skills deficits. Each of the subtypes has a brief description of characteristics, test performance, cause, and needs in therapy.

Auditory Decoding Deficit

Listening characteristics

- "Mishears" acoustic features of speech
- Trouble hearing in environments when the listener is not familiar with vocabulary, or when there are no contextual or visual cues to help, or when there is excess noise/reverberation, or in group listening situation
- Says "I can't hear"; requests lots of repeats
- Tends to be slow and inaccurate in responding

Language characteristics

- May exhibit difficulties in acquiring appropriate first- or second-language vocabulary, use of morphologic markers and semantic skills including multiple meaning words
- Poor reading decoding, and spelling; does not spell phonetically

Test performance

- Markedly poor performance on tests of degraded speech
- Poor on auditory closure tasks; errors are phonemically similar to target
- Bilateral deficits on dichotic listening tasks
- Manifests like sensorineural hearing loss
- Poorer verbal than performance IQ
- Tends to perform more poorly on word- or name-memory tests than memory-for-sentences
- Poor performance on auditory discrimination (e.g., TAPS)
- Does not spell phonetically
- Speech sound discrimination problems
- Many say this is the classic profile of (C)APD

Causes

- Poor neural representation of acoustic-phonetic features of speech
- Auditory cortex involvement; bilateral problem
- Site of dysfunction: thalamocortical pathways and/or primary auditory cortex

Needs in listening skills training

- Consonant-vowel discrimination
- Auditory closure activities to teach contextual cues
- Auditory training and noise tolerance training
- Lipreading exercises
- Critical listening activities

Needs in language therapy

- Word association, categorization, and labeling
- Vocabulary building
- Work on reading and spelling
- Phonemic training and auditory closure activities

Suggestions for classroom

- Improve acoustic access to information
- Preferential seating
- Auditory trainer
- Preteach new information
- Teacher repetition of information but rephrasing confuses the student
- Add visual cues

Compensatory activities

- Assertiveness training
- Identify adverse listening situations

Prosodic Deficit

Listening characteristics

- May misunderstand what other students say

Language characteristics

- May be a monotonic speaker or reader
- Pragmatic language problems: may misinterpret intent of communications and react inappropriately or with hurt feelings; doesn't "get" jokes or sarcasm
- Receptive language problems related to difficulty interpreting suprasegmental aspects of language (e.g., problems understanding heteronyms, words that change meaning as a function of stress such as CONvict vs. convict
- Poor sight word recognition but good decoders. They try to apply a phonological approach to reading

- Decreased reading rate and comprehension
- Decreased spelling and writing
- Math calculations difficulties
- Other: may not be adept at art or music; has decreased visual skills and has visual figure-ground problems

Test performance

- Not a true auditory processing problem because the right hemisphere is a source of the problem
- Poor left ear scores for dichotic listening tasks with difficulty humming tonal patterns and verbally labeling them on temporal patterning tasks
- Decreased pattern perception
- May score within normal on all speech/language tests, but something is "just a little off"

Causes

- Inefficient function in nonprimary, or right hemisphere
- Bilateral deficits on tests of temporal patterning in verbal report and humming conditions
- Left ear deficits on dichotic speech tasks

Needs in listening skills training

- Pattern recognition activities
- Prosody training: recognition and use of rhythm, stress and intonation patterns in speech
- Music and nonspeech rhythm perception

Needs in language therapy

- Symbolic and/or nonverbal language skills
- Social communication skills
- Reading aloud daily with exaggerated prosody

Suggestions for classroom

- Needs an animated teacher with modified voice using lots of demonstration and examples
- Needs experiential, well-structured, hands-on learning environment

- Information needs to be repeated with emphasis on key words and altered pacing
- Use visual cues

Compensatory activities

- Encourage music and dance
- Key word extraction

Integration Deficit

Listening characteristics

- Significant difficulty in noise not due to reduced redundancy
- Difficulty localizing/tracking a moving sound
- Says the right ear is "better" over binaural hearing aids

Language characteristics

- Frequently complain they don't know how to do tasks
- May have syntactic, semantic, and pragmatic problems
- Receptive language problems for complex or lengthy auditory-verbal messages
- Difficulty labeling
- Other: may have a variety of auditory, multimodality integration, and learning-related problems; may perform more poorly when required to look and listen (e.g., when taking notes)

Test performance

- Signal/noise problem
- Left ear deficit on dichotic speech tasks combined with bilateral deficits on tests of temporal patterning in linguistic labeling condition
- Poor labeling of temporal patterns
- Does better on patterning tasks when asked to hum patterns heard

Cause

- Inefficient function in corpus callosum

Needs in listening skills training

- To improve message understanding, teach student to repeat the message verbatim with associate visual cues or example rather than rephrasing

Needs in language therapy

- Label tactile stimuli for instance have the student reach into a bag and describe what she or he is feeling
- Activities that start with "whole" and then teach "parts-to-whole" skills

Suggestions for classroom

- Reduce or avoid use of multimodality cues
- Provide a note taker
- Have a well structured environment
- Allow extra time for assignments and tests
- Allow the student to take tests in a separate, quiet room

Compensatory activities

- Avoid division of attention
- Other: Possibly sensory integration therapy
- Encourage music and/or dance lessons

Remediation of Listening Skills Deficits

Although the underlying cause of the problem may vary, children with APD and/or SLI and/or LLD need to work on developing listening skills. According to the ASHA (2005) report:

> Treatment and management goals are determined on the basis of diagnostic test findings, the individual's case history, and related speech-language and psychoeducational assessment data, should focus both on remediation of deficit skills and management of the disorder's impact on the individual. (p. 11)

To this end, three approaches are suggested by ASHA to be implemented simultaneously when appropriate: *direct skills remediation, compensatory strategies,* and *environmental modifications* (ASHA, 2005, p. 11). As stated in the ASHA report,

> Computerized delivery offers the advantages of multisensory stimulation in an engaging format that provides generous feedback and reinforcement . . . despite the potential of computerized approaches additional data are needed to demonstrate the effectiveness and efficacy of these approaches. (p.11)

The following summarizes recommendations contained in the ASHA 2005 (pp 11–12) report under the three headings mentioned above.

Direct Skills Remediation (Auditory Training)

Direct skills remediation involves bottom-up training to alter auditory behavior. These activities may include but are not limited to procedures targeting:

- intensity, frequency, and duration discrimination
- phoneme discrimination and phoneme-to-grapheme skills
- temporal gap discrimination
- temporal ordering or sequencing
- pattern recognition
- localization/lateralization
- recognition of auditory information presented within a background of noise or competition

Other activities to increase interhemispheric transfer of information to enhance binaural hearing and binaural processing including but not limited to:

- exercises using interaural temporal offsets and intensity differences
- unimodal exercises (e.g., linking prosodic and linguistic acoustic features)

■ multimodal exercises (e.g., writing to dictation, verbally describing a picture while drawing)

Compensatory Strategies

Compensatory strategies involve top-down treatment approaches designed to minimize the impact of the residual (C)APD that is not resolved through auditory training and that interacts and exacerbates deficits in other language, cognitive, and academic areas:

■ strengthening higher order central resources such as language, memory, attention
■ metalinguistic strategies including schema induction and discourse cohesion devices, context-derived vocabulary building, phonological awareness, and semantic network expansion
■ metacognitive strategies include self-instruction, cognitive problem solving, and assertiveness training
■ motivation and a sense of self-efficacy are crucial to successful intervention

Environmental Modifications

Environmental modifications include both bottom-up (enhancing signal and listening environment) and top-down (classroom, instructional, workplace, recreational, and home accommodations) management approaches:

■ Environmental accommodations to enhance listening environment may include but are not limited to:
(1) preferential seating
(2) use of visual aids
(3) reduction of competing signals and reverberation time
(4) use of assistive listening systems based on the student's profile of auditory processing deficits. (See ASHA report page 12 for specific recommendations)
(5) advising speakers to speak more slowly, pause more often, and emphasize key words

■ Enhancing the student's ability to access communication and learning within the classroom and at home:

(1) focused listening: use of note takers, preview questions, organizers

(2) redundancy: multisensory instruction, computer mediation

(3) use of written output such as E-mail and mind-maps

The ASHA report concluded with suggested outcome measures:

■ indices of auditory performance such as pattern tests, dichotic digits, speech recognition for time-compressed speech

■ functional indices of metalanguage such as phonemic analysis, phonemic synthesis

■ more global measures of listening and communication such as self-assessment for informant communication and education scales (p. 13).

Let's Get Practical

To help the student or practitioner move to implementation of the above discussion, the following *selected goals* are suggested to increase a student's listening skills only. The goals for Compensatory Strategies and Environmental Modifications will not be covered in this chapter. The goals are presented as Long-Term Goals with Short-Term Objectives. If you work in a setting using other terms, you can substitute those. For instance, in many school districts, Long-Term Goals are referred to as Standards and Short-Term Objectives are referred to as Benchmarks.

Direct Listening Skills (Auditory) Training

Long-Term Goal: Increase the student's listening skills through enhancing intensity, frequency, and duration discrimination. Ferre (2007) explained that "in auditory discrimination training, the goal is to improve the listener's ability to discriminate, identify, and recognize fine and/or rapidly changing acoustic cues" (p. 189).

Short-Term Objective: Increase the student's listening skills through increased ability to recognize and identify similarities and differences in isolated speech sounds presented orally by the clinician.

Example: "/b/ /g/ are those the same or different?"

Short-Term Objective: Increase the student's listening skills through increased ability to identify if words presented orally by the clinician begin or end with the same or different sound.

Example: " 'soup,' 'salad,' do those begin with the same or different sounds?"

Example: " 'cat,' 'cap,' do those end with the same or different sounds?"

Short-Term Objective: Increase the student's listening skills through increased ability to identify if the vowels in two CVC monosyllabic words are the same or different.

Example: " 'tip,' 'top,' do those have the same or different middle sounds?"

Suggested Materials

- Any list of words (e.g., *40,000 Selected Words*, Block-colsky, Frazer, & Frazer, 1987),
- Phonological awareness materials such as *Sourcebooks of Phonological Awareness Training* (Goldsworthy, 1998, 2000; Goldsworthy & Pieretti, 2004).
- Treating Auditory Processing Difficulties (Sloan, 1986)
- Lindamood Bell Phoneme Sequencing Program (LiPS)
- Using some of the existing computerized programs, although the data concerning these are not always conclusive. Ferre (2007) suggested the following:
  - FastForward (http://www.fastforward.com)
  - Earobics (Cognitive Concepts, 1997, 1998) for 4- to 7-year-olds including six interactive games (http://www.earobics.com)
  - SoundSmart (Sanford, 2001). Ross-Swain and Geffner (2009) explained that this software program for 4-year-olds through adult increases auditory attention

through building phonemic awareness, listening skills, working memory, mental processing speed, and self-control.

■ Captain's Log (http://www.braintrain.com), a program for children and adults, recommended by Ross-Swain & Geffner (2009). The Attention module includes a series of pitch, patterns and discrimination activities.

Long-Term Goal: Increase the student's listening skills through temporal gap discrimination.

Bellis (2003) described Keith's (2000) random Gap Detection Test involving brief tones of octave frequencies from 250 to 4000 Hz presented in pairs with a silent interval between each pair. Listeners are required to indicate whether they hear one stimulus or two. The gap detection threshold is defined as the smallest interval at which the listener consistently identifies two stimuli (p. 210).

Long-Term Goal: Increase the student's listening skills through increased pattern recognition.

Ferre (2007) suggested formal therapeutic activities not always available to student clinicians and practitioners. The following activities she described are more available (p. 190).

Short-Term Objective: Increase the student's listening skills through imitating rhythmic patterns (e.g., long-short-long through tapping the response).

Example: clinician taps different patterns on table or drum and student is to imitate.

Short-Term Objective: Increase the student's listening skills through imitating tonal patterns (e.g., high-low-high through humming the response).

Example: clinician hums various patterns and the student is to imitate.

Ferre suggested carryover activities through some informal games including Mad Gab, Bop It, Simon Says (p. 190).

Long-Term Goal: Increase the student's listening skills through increased ability to localize/lateralize sound.

Bellis (2003) described formalized localization training that is often unavailable to student clinicians or practitioners.

Activities: Bellis also suggested the well known children's games such as "Blind Man Bluff" and "Marco Polo" as informal activities to train sound localization abilities "These games can provide an excellent opportunity for generalization of localization abilities in real-world listening environments in a fun, entertaining manner, especially for young children" (p. 365).

Long-Term Goal: Increase the student's listening skills through recognition of auditory information presented within a background of noise or competition.

Activities: Goldsworthy (2003) suggested the following:

- Tape-record various background noises such as cafeteria noise or classroom noise, and play a tape while you ask the student to follow a variety of sequential directions presented orally
- teach the student to identify noisy environments that are difficult for him or her and what needs to be done to alter the environment

Geffner and Ross-Swain (2008) suggested doing this activity using high interest figure (verbally presented information) with low interest background and then reverse this to low interest figure and high interest background

Example: high-interest figure: something the student is interested in; low- interest background: white noise; low interest figure: something irrelevant to the student; high-interest background: a song or movie of high interest to the student.

Long-Term Goal: Increase the student's listening skills through increased interhemispheric transfer of information to enhance binaural hearing and binaural processing including but not limited to:

Short-Term Objective: Increase the student's listening skills through having him or her carry out opposing directives such as telling him or her to take two steps forward and he or she has to do the opposite (i.e., take two steps backward) (Geffner & Ross-Swain, 2008).

Long-Term Goal: Increase the student's listening skills through multimodal exercises.

Short-Term Objective: Increase the student's listening skills through phoneme-to-grapheme skills.

Example: The student will print the grapheme (letter) corresponding to the phoneme (speech sound) verbally presented by the clinician.

Suggested Materials

- Any list of words (e.g., *40,000 Selected Words*, Blockcolsky et al., 1987)
- Phonological awareness materials such as *Sourcebooks of Phonological Awareness Training* (Goldsworthy, 1998, 2000; Goldsworthy & Pieretti, 2004).
- Treating Auditory Processing Difficulties (Sloan, 1986)
- Lindamood Bell Phoneme Sequencing Program (LiPS)

Short-Term Objective: The student will increase listening skills through the multimodality exercise of writing to dictation. The clinician can verbally dictate the words, phrases, or sentences to be written by the student.

Suggested Materials: Any book

Short-Term Objective: The student will increase listening skills through the multimodality exercise of verbally describing a picture while drawing.

Suggested Materials: Any draw-and-tell book or exercise, for instance see Thompson (1990) *Draw and Tell* book.

Short-Term Objective: The student will increase listening skills through verbal-to-motor transfer through having the student find specific objects or shapes with the left hand from a grab bag or behind a screen (i.e., the student cannot see the objects/shapes) (Bellis, 2003).

Short-Term Objective: The student will increase listening skills through what Bellis (2003) suggested as a motor-to-verbal transfer that occurs when the above is reversed: student finds objects with the left hand and is instructed to label and verbally describe them by shape, texture, identification, and so forth.

Long-Term Goal: Increase the student's listening skills through unimodal exercises (linking prosodic and linguistic acoustic features).

Short-Term Objective: Increase the student's listening skills through auditory closure tasks requiring the student to predict missing word. Ferre (2007) explained that these top-down activities target the ability to predict a missing target sound or word based upon context.

Example: Ferre (2007) recommended beginning with familiar materials and moving toward more linguistically challenging materials (p. 193):

- nursery rhymes (e.g., Humpty Dumpty sat on a _____)
- predictable everyday sentences (e.g., When we go to the library, we can get _____)
- more challenging (e.g., Don't let the cat out of the _____)
- more challenging: specific parts of speech omitted: (e.g., The pitcher _____ the ball to the catcher).
- predicting targets with a missing syllable: (e.g., wall-____-per)
- predicting missing sound (e.g., s-p-____ch) (answer: long E sound

Short-Term Objective: Increase the student's listening skills through use of discourse cohesion devices (learning to "key in" to tag words and conjunctions).

Example: training the student to signal when hearing "tag" words such as: first, last, next, before, after

Example: training the student to signal when hearing conjunctions such as: and, but, after, either, because, if, however, rather than

Short-Term Objective: Increase the student's listening skills through use of prosody. According to Ferre (2007), prosody training "improves the listener's ability to attach meaning to the prosodic or suprasegmental aspects of speech, including melody, rhythm, timing, and emphasis" (p. 193).

Example: training the student to recognize sarcasm (e.g., Now THAT was cute!)"

Example: training the student to recognize changes in meaning based on stress or intonation (e.g., declarative: Stop. interrogative Stop? Or exclamatory STOP! (Ferre, 2007, p. 193).

Example: training the student to practice using heteronyms, or words that change meaning depending upon stress pattern (e.g., OBject versus obJECT) (Ferre, 2007, p. 193).

The purpose of this chapter was to review and highlight the work on Listening Skills in Children. Terms including (central) auditory processing disorders, specific language impairment, and language-learning disabilities were highlighted to emphasize the overlap in symptomatology among the descriptions. Goals of listening skills included in the ASHA (2005) Technical Report on Auditory Processing Disorders were included with suggested terminology for inclusion in clinical reports as well as suggested targets and materials. Chapter 4 will present the rationale for the oral-written language strand.

Remember: Your client may need to have *listening skills* targeted as the first strand to include in his or her language therapy. She or he may demonstrate the need to return to the earlier *play* strand, *or* she or he may need to revisit the listening skills strand while working on later strands. He or she may now be ready to go on to the *oral-written language* strand.

Chapter 4

Early Oral-Written Language: The Rationale

*T*he purpose of this chapter is not to review the causes and consequences of childhood language disorders. Likewise, this chapter does not review the myriad philosophies of how to increase oral and written language or present the many evidence-based programs and practices that exist to work with children who are delayed or impaired in the development of an oral-written language system. As mentioned previously, in keeping with the overall intent of this resource, I embrace the analogy of language acquisition as a French braid proposed by Dickinson and McCabe (1991):

> The process of language acquisition can be thought of as being like a French braid rather than as a sequential process. Like a braid, language consists of multiple strands: phonology, semantics, syntax, discourse, reading, and writing-that are picked up at various times and woven in with the other strands to create a beautiful whole. (p. 1)

The purpose of this chapter is to explain the rationale behind the particular approach I have developed to work with young children with delayed or disordered oral-written language development. The "how-tos" of linking the strands of language and literacy are covered in Chapter 5. To move us in that direction, this chapter covers the following topics:

- ■ Where do goals come from in child language therapy?
- ■ What are some guiding principles in therapy? This section focuses on" the linguistic innateness theory; the theory of neurolinguistic development; humans as pattern seekers,

and the concept of goodness of fit; and implicit and explicit teaching.
- Why do clients need to work on these goals?
- What materials should be used?

Where Do Goals Come From in Child Language Therapy?

Historically, speech and language specialists have been taught to "divide" language into receptive and expressive skills. Traditional training programs have taught students of speech-language pathology to parse up skills, to divide language into discrete behaviors. Damico (1988) and Kent (1990) are among those who advised against the fragmentation fallacy that results when language is analyzed into separate domains such as phonology, semantics, syntax, and pragmatics. Although the tests we administer as SLPs divide language into these domains, it is up to the interventionist to meld the fragments into bigger units and bring them to an automatic skill level. If we divide language into "bits" and leave them unintegrated without weaving the strands of that braid together, the results of our labor may be tantamount to Humpty Dumpty after the fall. Although I certainly value the current tests we use in child language clinics, I also am guarded as to where the test results lead practitioners.

Among the areas in speech-language pathology that have evolved exponentially over the past years is child language disorders. One of the purposes of existing assessment tools is to define and delimit the problem areas with which our clients present. But, as test users, we must be ever vigilant as to the specific language domains and test items that were selected by test authors to be included in the tests we administer. There needs to be some kind of a match between the test author(s)' notion of what is important in child language with what the test user believes is important. One test author may choose to look at basic concepts such as "categories" or "opposites" in a test, and another author may select to assess developing semantics/vocabulary. Two different test authors may choose to "zero in" on syntactic/morphologic aspects of language and look at very different items. One author may include items to assess verbs, prepositions, adjectives, and so forth; another may examine the child's use of past tense forms, possessives, and pronouns. Although all are important areas to assess and, if needed, to include in a client's remedial plan, if we allow the test to narrow our vision of the child's overall language needs, we provide "piece-meal" therapy. Unless we keep the big picture in our minds, we compartmentalize the child's overall language system and offer a limited range of services. We target "language piece" by "language piece" and, hopefully, include enough isolated bits of language in our remedial program to move the child toward acquiring an elaborate language system. How often do practitioners, especially student clinicians, target specific syntactic targets, for instance, to increase the use of "he/she" pronouns, or to increase the use of present progressive –"ing"? Student clinicians target specific items such as these for approximately 12 weeks of therapy during an academic semester and post-test at the end of the semester. Many times students are pleased that their client's performance has increased on the readministered test, but disappointed to hear their client revert to use of "old structures" outside the therapy room. If you are working with a client who presents with isolated needs, this approach certainly is one to consider. The child who needs work, for instance, adding past tense markers, or increasing vocabulary, and so on, an approach targeting only those needs may be sufficient. But, if you are talking about children with more extensive language needs, you will drastically limit your remedial attempts if you target only specific semantic/syntactic goals included in existing language assessment tools.

In many ways, I am talking about the same kind of rationale that underlies "articulation therapy" versus "phonological processes therapy." The more traditional "articulation" approach targets one or two sounds at a time, usually in the initial, final, and then medial position of words, prior to carryover into phrases, sentences, and finally conversational speech. In the "phonological processes" approach, processes, not specific speech sounds, are targeted. Advocates of this approach believe that immersing a client into various phonological processes that include more than one speech sound at a time through auditory bombardment and specific instruction on production is more far reaching than the traditional sound-by sound articulation approach. Rather, the process of front sounds (/m/, /p/, and /b)/, for example, are highlighted so the client learns about "frontness" rather than how to produce three separate speech sounds. Rather than learning how to produce the specific words used to stimulate awareness of /b/ words, or /m/ words, or /p/ words, the client emerges with a more general understanding of how to produce many words beginning with "front" sounds. The approach to stimulating a "process" rather than "specific sounds" should result in knowledge about how to produce a number of sounds included within that process. Tyler, Edwards, and Saxman (1987) explained that

> the major assumption of a phonological process-based treatment approach is that remediation is maximized through generalization that occurs across the sounds affected by a particular process when only a few sounds undergoing that process are taught. It is assumed that the elimination of a few specific sound errors produces change in the underlying process accounting for those errors. (p. 393)

Targeting only isolated syntactic constructions in a child who needs many syntactic-morphologic constructions falls short of the mark. In this unidirectional approach to language therapy, the clinician selects the target to be remediated, chooses the picture cards that depict the construction, models the construction, for example, "The boy is walking," The girl is talking" and so forth, and asks the client to repeat what has been said. This approach is so "clinician directed!" Unless this clinician specifically builds in experiences during therapy sessions where the client generates a need to use and *create* the syntactic form, in this case, present progressive, he or she may exit a therapy session and a semester of therapy sessions still weak in generating the language necessary to convey his or her wants and needs. Unidirectional therapy (i.e., from the clinician's "head" to the child's "head") simply misses the mark. The clinician creates, the client "robotically" repeats without really *generating* the construction(s) needed to communicate his or her needs.

I talk with my student clinicians about my notion of "the slot theory" in child language therapy. Like the "processes" approach to speech sound production improvement, "slot theory" thinking lends itself to the notion of teaching, for example, about "adjectiveness" rather than selecting specific "colors" or "sizes" or "shapes" the client misses on a given language test. If a client misses test items indicating a weakness in the use of adjectives, don't just teach those specific items. Instead of isolating these specific words, teach the client about adjectives through bombarding him or her with many kinds of adjectives. If the client misses a color name on a test, more than likely she or he has some problems using a number of adjectives. Stated differently, unless this client has had limited or no exposure to a certain adjective, she or he probably has difficulty or is delayed with many adjectives, not just that specific adjective. More than likely, the problem is not just with that part of speech called an adjective, but the difficulty with the semantic relations referred to as "modifiers." Rather than treat this child by teaching the specific color names missed on the test, select a number of adjectives (modifiers) to expand the noun phrase. Rather than targeting one color adjective, "red," to describe the noun "car," (if the client missed the modifier "red" on a test), I propose using many different color words, "red, blue, yellow, green," and so forth, as well as many size words, "big, little, medium, huge, teeny." Likewise, introduce shape words, such as "round, square, rectangular, or triangular." During play with the cars, you can now label the car as a "red car" or "big car" or "rectangular car." Or you can talk about the "big, red, rectangular car." Like the processes approach, the more the child is bombarded with "adjectiveness," the more likely he or she will begin "marking the slot" for adjectives. He or she may describe the "red car" in one instance and the "big car" in another, and the "big, red car" in yet another. The child has learned to modify the noun through the use of adjectives. My experience has taught me that, once that "slot" is opened for adjectives, the client will go on to fill the "adjective bin" with lots of useful modifiers. You no longer have to teach one adjective after another because the test identifies those as missing or emerging. You open the "modifier slot" and the client will begin to fill the slot with many adjectives and in time with adjectives you didn't teach.

Think About This: As I point out to my student clinicians, if a client is having problems with any of the above, we need to be asking the question: why does she or he have this problem? Teaching specific "adjective words," or any other part(s) of speech or semantic relations, is tantamount to providing "band-aid therapy." This kind of therapy is useful only in putting out "small fires." If that's all the client needs to work on, terrific! Teach the specific word(s) and let it go. But this is not a language delay or disorder. When the symptoms are pervasive, teaching specific words is not going to get "to the heart of the problem." We need to determine what the underlying cause of the language problem or delay is. This takes us back to our introductory courses in child language disorders. Does this child have a hearing loss? Is there an emotional component? Is there a cognitive deficit? Is he or she a twin? Is there a good model for this child to imitate in the environment? Or has this child gotten stuck somewhere in the stages Jon Locke describes? (see the next section in this chapter, Guiding Principles of Therapy). Has this child been accumulating words but somehow fallen behind in separating the holophrases (e.g., "shoesnsox") into single words (shoes and sox)? Has this child somehow not learned about "word juncture," where one word ends and the next one begins? Rather than teach isolated bits of language, do we need to help the language acquisition device get "ignited?" (see the next section in this chapter, Guiding Principles of Therapy). Do we need to help the holophrases move on to become "chopped up?" If we search for the root of the problem, we then add in work to help with the underlying problem and our overall language remediation program works faster and more efficiently. The specific items missed on language tests provide us with a list of symptoms of how the language problem manifests itself but not with the underlying reason for the problem. We must continue to search for the underlying reason for the problem and treat that as well.

Let us look at some specific examples from two current widely used child language assessment tools. One tool used particularly in the public school setting is the Clinical Evaluation of Language Fundamentals-4 (Semel, Wiig, & Secord, 2003). The authors explained that the subtest Word Structure assesses "the student's ability to (a) apply word structure rules (morphology) to mark inflections, derivations, and comparisons; and (b) select and use appropriate pronouns to refer to people, objects, and possessive relationships" (p. 22). Included among the assessed items are: regular plurals (books, horses); irregular plurals (mice, children); third person singular (reads, flies); and possessive nouns (Paula's boot, king's/queen's). The authors explained that the subtest Formulated Sentences assesses "the student's ability to formulate complete, semantically and grammatically correct spoken sentences of increasing length and complexity (i.e., simple, compound, and complex sentences), using given words such as car, if because, and contextual constraints imposed by illustrations" (p. 33). In the Formulated Sentences subtest, using a picture the examiner tells a young client, "Here is a picture of children in a library. I will use the word *book* in a sentence to talk about this picture. *The girl is reading a book.* Or I could say, *"That book is on the table."* Following trial items, the client is to make up sentences that go with the pictures shown using certain stimulus words including, but not limited to: children, forgot, always, car, best, third, quickly, neither, however, as soon as, in order to, even though, as a consequence. Finally, in the Concepts and Following Directions subtest of the CELF-4, the authors explained that the purpose of the subtest is "to evaluate the student's ability to (a) interpret spoken directions of increasing length and complexity containing concepts that require logical operations; (b) remember the names, characteristics, and order of mention of objects; and (c) identify from among several choices the pictured objects that were mentioned" (p. 18). Some examples from the test include: "Point to the third big car;" "point to the fourth black ball and the first white ball;" "point to the big black apple, the little fish, and the little white apple;" "point to the ball and the fish before you point to the shoe and the apple;" "point to the shoe and the ball after you point to the big fish and the little black fish."

Another widely used assessment tool for young children is the Preschool Language Scale-Fourth edition (PLS-4) (Zimmerman, Steiner, & Pond, 2002). The following two test items were selected to illustrate Auditory Comprehension:

Item 34, which is included in the 36- to 41-month level: Understands pronouns using stimuli from the Picture Manual.

Practice: Look at these children. They are wearing shoes. Show me *his* shoes. Show me *her* shoes.

  a. Look at these two children. Show me *her* hat.
  b. Show me *his* hat.
  c. Look at these children. Show me *her* jacket.
  d. Show me *his* jacket.
  e. Now look at these pictures. Find the one that shows:
  f. *She* is on the stairs.
  g. Now find: *He* is in the pool.

Item 48, which is included in the 54- to 59-month level: Understands noun + two modifying adjectives using Picture Manual.

Practice: I want you to look at all of the dogs. Find the *big brown* dog.

a. Point to the *small black* dog.
b. Point to the *big white* dog.

The following two test items were selected to illustrate Expressive Communication:

Item 51, which is included in the 54- to 59-month level: Uses qualitative concepts *short* and *long* using pictures from the Manual.

Practice: Look at these pictures. This chain is long; this chain is _____.

a. This dress is short; this dress is _____ (long)
b. Her ribbons are long; her ribbons are _____ (short)
c. This rope is short; this rope is _____ (long)

Item 54, which is included in the 54- to 59-month level: Uses past tense forms using stimuli from the Picture Manual.

Practice: Look at these pictures. The girl is skating. Now she has finished. Tell me what she did. She _____.

a. Right now she is washing her hands. Now she has finished. Tell me what she did. She _____.
b. In this picture the ice cream is melting. Tell me what happened to the ice cream in this picture. It _____.

Student clinicians learn to administer assessment tools such as these and "get lured"into writing goals targeting specific items as highlighted above. Our assessment tools lead us almost necessarily to specific goals, which, in and of itself, is not a bad thing, but if left unintegrated into the child's overall oral-written language system, then where does it go? What does it tie into? Although taught not to "teach to any test," students and practitioners in child language therapy frequently target specific "parts of speech" or "basic concepts," zeroing in on specific items that may have been included among items missed on assessment tools. Clinicians then write goals and objectives or standards and benchmarks to include in their client(s)' plan(s) aimed primarily at the specific items missed on the assessment tools.

Stop and Go Back to What I Asked Several Pages Ago: What is the underlying cause of the problem? Why is your client experiencing difficulty acquiring the specified items in the first place? *What else is needed* in your overall remedial program that will help your client generalize faster and be more successful in acquiring a mature language system sooner? Does your client need to link back to the play strand? (see Chapter 2). What about adding in several goals included in the listening strand? (see Chapter 3). Is it time to move into early literacy in print through beginning reading and writing? (see Chapter 5).

A wonderful source to help us to identify specific goals and objectives was produced by Nelson (1990). This is a gold mine of information that is relevant for both beginning and seasoned child language clinicians. I'll list several goals and objectives here to illustrate. My newer, evolved, approach is to be sure to help my students to understand these goals cannot just be considered as isolated goals. Rather, they need to be woven back into the patchwork quilt of the child's overall oral-written language system, that is, through *verbally producing* the needed vocabulary words and/or syntactic constructions, through *reading* the same vocabulary words and/or syntactic constructions in books and through *writing* the same vocabulary and/or syntactic constructions into more and more complex written language. A few examples from Nelson's book follow:

Information Processing: Early Language: One-Word Utterances

Goal: The child will use one-word utterances to communicate sentence-like meanings (holophrases) to others in the environment.

Short-Term Objectives: The child will

1. Use gestures to request, reject, or identify objects/people/animals in a structured play situation (at least five gestures used communicatively in each of two consecutive interactions).
2. Indicate word comprehension by looking at, pointing to, picking up, or giving an adult objects/people/animals

named, or preparing for action (as in b below), in a structured play context, with minimal contextual support and not gestural or gaze cues from the adult (word recognition on three out of four trials each for at least two words in each of the following categories):

a. name of family member or pet (Mommy, Fish)
b. label for game or social ritual (byebye, peek-a-boo)
c. manipulable object/toy (blanket, telephone, shoe)
d. body parts (hair, nose, belly button)
e. food related (cookie, bottle)

Information Processing: Basic Sentences

Goal: The child will use basic sentence constructions to communicate a variety of meanings to other persons in the environment.

Short-Term Objectives: The child will

1. demonstrate comprehension of the following semantic cases and verb types in (NP) + VP constructions spoken by the speech-language pathologist by pointing to objects/pictures or performing an action (4 of 5 trials correct on 9 of 13 types for two consecutive sessions):
   a. semantic cases
      (1) agentive [pronoun or noun "doer" of action] (baby is crying.)
      (2) experiencer [pronoun or noun subject of a state verb] (The boy feels happy.)
      (3) dative [indirect object] (Give Mommy a kiss.)
      (4) objective [direct object affected by action] (Push the truck.)
      (5) factitive [direct object resulting from action] (Let's make cookies.)
      (6) instrumental [prepositional phrase indicating object used for performing action] (Hit it with the hammer.)
      (7) locative [prepositional or adverbial phrase] (Put them in the oven. Come here.]
      (8) possessor [person or object owning something or exhibiting a train] (Put it in Mommy's purse. Where's the bear's tail?)

(9) Modifier [adjective, article, demonstrative pronoun, quantifier, or prepositional phrase] (Bring me the big ball. I want that one. He needs lots of modeling clay. She's the girl with curly hair.)

Another outstanding source to use for selecting and writing goals is the *IEP Companion* (Wilson, Lanza, & Evans 2005). Stepped out differently than Nelson's (described above), the IEP companion selects a training target and a yearly goal, then coordinates Individual Objectives with Classroom Objectives. This source moves more toward what I am suggesting in this resource by targeting goals in oral language and then reading and writing. The section on Possessives was chosen to illustrate here. Not all the individual and classroom objectives have been listed.

Yearly Goal: to develop correct use of possessive nouns in conversation and in writing.

Individual Objective: Imitates the instructor's model as she labels possessions, like "Kim's" or "Raoul's."

Corresponding Intervention Objective: During a group time activity, imitates the model that states ownership of each child's possessions. ("This is Jennifer's crayon.")

Individual Objective: Locates objects described. ("Find David's shirt.")

Corresponding Intervention Objective: After listening to directions using students' names, locates the objects described. ("Show me Brianna's desk.")

Individual Objective: Answers questions about possessions using possessive nouns in single words. ("Whose is this?" *"Lynette's."*)

Corresponding Intervention Objective: During an activity like snack time, answers questions using single possessive nouns. ("Whose cracker is this?" *"Laura's."*)

Individual Objective: Labels objects in pictures as requested using possessive nouns in short phrases. (The firefighter's hat.")

Corresponding Intervention Objective: While talking about lesson-related pictures, answers questions with possessive nouns in short phrases. (Whose dog ran away in the story?" *"Miguel's dog."*)

Individual Objective: Writes possessive nouns in short phrases to name objects and pictures requested. (*"Matthew's pencil."*)

Corresponding Intervention Objective: During a classroom activity, writes possessive nouns in short phrases for objects and pictures requested. ("What is this?" *"The teacher's desk."*)

Individual Objective: Corrects a written paragraph by changing inappropriately used possessive nouns.

Corresponding Intervention Objective: After reading a paragraph from a classroom lesson that has been altered, rewrites the paragraph correcting possessive nouns. (*"The dog's eyes were shining."*)

Individual Objective: Writes a sentence using possessive nouns to describe surroundings. (*"The book's cover is red."*)

Corresponding Intervention Objective: After participating in a classroom activity, writes sentences using possessive nouns to describe the activity. (*"Mark's opinion was not the same as Nathan's."*)

Individual Objective: Uses possessive nouns to relate personal life experiences.

Corresponding Intervention Objective: During a small group discussion, tells about family members using possessive nouns. (*"My mother's name is Renee. I have two sisters. One's name is Bianca and the other one's name is Jessica."*)

Individual Objective: Uses possessive nouns to write a story.

Corresponding Intervention Objective: During a classroom lesson, uses possessive nouns in a written report about a current event. ("Summarize the magazine article you read about the scientist's discovery.")

Over the years my students and coworkers have agreed that, although the above type sources are extremely helpful in moving from test results to selection of goals and in writing goals, the following questions invariably arise: So now what? And what is this tied to? What do we do with this information? Now how do we teach/implement our selected goals? What does this particular goal have to do with the rest of what this client needs to do in school? Before turning to specific suggestions on linking the strands of language and literacy in Chapter 5, the rest of this chapter highlights some guiding principles to consider in child language therapy.

What Are Some Guiding Principles in Therapy?

Like other students of speech-language pathology, I have learned the various theoretical accounts of what is involved in language acquisition. The reader is directed toward one recent summary by Nelson (2010) for a number of important theoretical accounts of how young children acquire language. After having worked with hundreds of children with language disorders and supervised hundreds more seen in Child Language Disorders Clinics in university training programs, I have zeroed in on a few guiding theoretical underpinnings of my own therapy. I offer them here now because I think they will help to guide students and practitioners in how to link the strands of language and literacy. The topics I will include here are:

- The linguistic innateness theory
- Jon Locke's theory of neurolinguistic development
- Humans as pattern seekers and goodness of fit
- Implicit and explicit teaching
- Using contextualized materials

The Linguistic Innateness Theory

One theoretical account of child language acquisition that makes most sense to me clinically is the linguistic innateness theory. Perhaps the best known of the theorists supporting linguistic innateness, Chomsky (1980), held that language is an innate faculty that we are born with, that we are born with a set of linguistic rules a universal grammar, and that language builds on this language acquisition device (LAD). Children produce sentences they have never heard before. As Nelson (2010) summarized, "Logical arguments of these theorists point to the paucity of input required for most children to induce highly mature language rules by age 5 years, at a time when they do not yet demonstrate the cognitive skills needed for inductive and analogical reasoning for more general purposes" (p. 59). Furthermore, my experience over the years has led me to embrace Bruner's (1981) notion of a language acquisition support system (LASS). Bruner argued that, although there may well be a LAD, the family and surrounding social network of the child make up the LASS. The LASS has gained in importance for me over years of observing children delayed in language acquisition be surrounded with family members who don't talk a lot. And I've wondered which came first here—low verbal child or low verbal adult? And I have concluded a little of both. A child modeling an adult who does not talk a lot does not have the best model to imitate. On the other hand, having a child who does not talk a lot to his or her parents/grandparents/siblings is probably not as satisfying to be around as a child who is verbally engaging. The child who is not understood well because of the way she or he formulates her or his speech sounds or the way she or he strings words together soon learns to take fewer and fewer risks in talking. It doesn't take long for a child to become discouraged with people in their environment saying "huh?" "what did you say?" "tell me that again." Conversely, it doesn't take long for a parent or sibling to become discouraged when communicating with the child with language delay or impairment, so they learn to limit their verbal interactions with each other. Over the years, numerous families with language impaired children enter our clinic waiting room and sit silently looking at books or eating their lunches without verbally interacting with each other. They check in with each other visually, acknowledging each other's presence in the room and perhaps occasional directives such as "don't drop crumbs" or "give me it," but there is not a lot of real conversation. Both LAD and LASS make great intuitive sense to me.

Theory of Neurolinguistic Development

I have promoted Locke's (1997) theory of neurolinguistic development for years. According to this theory, language develops in young children in four fixed, overlapping, sequential phases, which are briefly summarized here.

Phase I involves the infant learning to "get by" in his or her native language by learning to take turns vocally with partners; orient to or mimic prosody she or he hears, communicatively gesture (e.g., raising arms up to indicate "pick me up"), to imitate various speech patterns, and attempt to alter the mental activity of the people in their environment (e.g., different cries to indicate thirst, hunger, bedtime).

During *Phase II*, beginning around 5 to 6 months and lasting up to 20 months, the infant is busy acquiring and storing utterances, primarily in the form of "holophrases" (e.g., "Iloveyou," "shoesnsox"). This phase, which involves active processing and storage in the right hemisphere through its strength in prosodic memory, is essential for the semantic domain of the developing linguistic system.

According to Locke's *Phase III*, between 18 and 20 to 36 months, the typically developing child is busily chopping up the holophrases sent forward from Phase II. In learning how to break words up into syllables and syllables into phonemes, the child is learning where words begin and end (word juncture), as well as morphological rules, for instance, when to add plural -es (horse, horses), and the possessive marker -'s to indicate ownership (dad, dad's).

During *Phase IV*, occurring from 3 years on, the child is engaged in linguistically integrating and elaborating his or her developing linguistic system. This allows the child to develop an ever-increasing vocabulary and an intricate word storage system. Locke explained that, because there was structural analysis during phase III, the pressure is "off a holistic type of memory, thereby enabling the creation of larger and larger vocabularies, in which each of the individual entries is merely a unique recombination of a small set of phonemes" (p. 275). Immensely important to Locke's theory is the notion that these four phases must happen in sequence and on time and that, in typically developing children, this all happens from infancy through about 6 to 8 years of age. The infant learns a lot about human communication during Phase I. Then the right hemisphere must develop a large enough supply of holophrases during Phase II to send to the left hemisphere during Phase III where they will be segmented into smaller parts—words, syllables, and sounds.

Humans as Pattern Seekers and Goodness of Fit

I've mentioned several times in this book that I firmly believe in the notion that the brain is a pattern seeker. It searches for similarities and differences. It wants to make sense of complexities. It wants to simplify things as well as discover how the simplification fits into a bigger picture. In an excellent description of this process, Wallach and Miller (1988) proposed the following:

> Humans are pattern seekers. We look for relatedness, for connections. Because we are equipped with neurological systems limited in processing capacity, we search for ways to clump what we know into manageable chunks. These polymorphous chunks constitute what we know and how we know. They organize the knowledge structures that form the basis for the strategies we develop to incorporate new information. (p. 13)

The authors go on to explain that organizing involves the search for patterns. In the broadest sense, knowledge can be described as an ongoing search for regularities or patterns. What we know is a summary or abstraction of our actual experiences. The way we organize our experiences serves as the basis of our knowledge; knowledge structures, sometimes referred to as schema, provide regularities for what we know and for what we learn. Language is one example of information that is organized in an orderly, systematic whole; however, there are many ways to organize what and how we know (p. 14).

Wallach and Miller continue by explaining that a primary way in which children attempt to move toward connections in their developing language system, and a *guiding* force in my own therapy decision making has to do with the notion of *goodness of fit*. In learning to speak their native language, children are engaged in making their best guess imitating what they hear. During this process, they unknowingly move from conscious, controlled information processing to automatic processing and finally to a metalinguistic level where they will be able to reflect on language as an object. At this highest level, they no longer have to think about when to add "-ed" to make certain verbs past tense or when to add "-s" to a noun to make it plural (birds) versus when they have to add "-es" to other nouns to make them plural (buses). Wallach and Miller explained:

> Attending to incoming information, whether feelings, pictures, sounds, tastes, or other sensory impressions, involves goodness-of-fit analysis. Auditory perceptual errors made by young children demonstrate the goodness-of-fit principle. The child who says "Give us this day our jellybread," for 'give us this day our daily bread," is involved in a goodness-of-fit analysis. The child who in reciting the pledge of allegiance says "I pledge a legion to the flag," or "And to the Republic for Richard stands," does the same thing. He or she tries to fit something new into something already known. (p. 14)

We have all heard young children make the types of errors cited above in their attempt to master their language. Through the years, I've heard many of these and I'll add just a few to those mentioned above: Six-year-old Mato told me the school he went to was "Citadel of Fake" (meaning Faith); 8-year-old Sharon talked about using the "emote control on the TV;" Seven-year-old Graham told me he and his mom were going to build a gingerbread house with "graham crappers"; 7-year-old Gianna talked to me about "licklick." I asked if she meant "licorice" and she said "That's a weird word"; she also told me that her mom was scared of the "pimbulls on their walk." I corrected saying "you mean pitbulls" and she said *"whatever!"* This one must be quite popular as another client, 8-year-old Alexis, recently told me that her grandmother had to chase away the "pimple." Had she let it go at that I would have thought perhaps dear granny had a temporary skin condition. My client continued with "It was bad . . . the pimple tried to attack grandma" at which point I asked for clarification! "What do you mean the pimple tried to attack?" Exasperated with me Alexis said: "That dog *chased* my grandma" and once again "pit bull" was the culprit. Time after time, our clients teach us about what "word juncture" is all about—not knowing where one word stops and the next one begins. And it's all about goodness of fit. They are simply trying to make their best guess at what they think we have just said to them.

A primary guiding principle on how organizing strategies occur offered to us by Wallach and Miller (1988) has to do with bottom-up/ top-down processing. They explain that, as learners, we establish a preferred goodness-of fit analyzer in which we may engage in a cognitively driven, top-down strategy of identifying a general outline

—a gestalt—the big picture of something and then work to figure out the details that will validate our hunch (p. 20). These authors explained that "top-down processing is analogous to deductive thinking . . . (in which) one formulates a general hypothesis and infers specific outcomes on the basis of the general principle" (p. 20). Conversely, in bottom-up processing, the learner starts with the data or details and works toward the bigger picture. The authors noted that bottom-up processing "is analogous to inductive thinking . . . (involving) gathering examples and letting them accumulate until the goodness-of-fit analyzer can draw a general conclusion based on the accumulated and individual details" (p. 21).

Language acquisition requires both top-down and bottom-up learning. It would seem that as young children are attempting to model adult language, they are engaging in a top-down process, trying to make their best guess at what we are saying, adding more and more pieces as they move closer to our model. When learning to sound out what printed words "say," children are engaged in an abstract to concrete bottom-up processing as they learn to translate graphemes to phonemes and to synthesize phonemes into the sounds of words. When retelling a story after reading it, a child is engaged in concrete to abstract t bottom-up processing. They move from recalling concrete pieces of information heard in a story to incorporating these with abstract features including character, setting, a problem, a sequence of events, resolution of a problem, and an ending (see Chapters 5 and 6 and corresponding CD).

Implicit and Explicit Teaching

In Chapter 3, a review of symptomatology was presented for three very common diagnostic categories in the area of child language disorders: auditory processing disorders, specific language impairment, and language-specific language impairment. As Johnston (2006) noted, "children who don't talk get much less practice in listening. If they find the auditory world confusing, they may even choose not to listen" (p. 93). After years of practicing speech-language pathology, and particularly in child language delay and disorders, I have realized that *my job* in helping children to do *their job* of finding the "best fit" of matching their developing language system with the adult version is to provide them with the models and appropriate materials. To that end, I want to submerge a client in materials where she or he can begin to discover patterns to make a best fit—to more closely approximate the adult model of speech and it is here that top-down/bottom-up processing meets implicit/explicit ways of teaching.

For 30 years, cognitive psychologist Reber (1996) studied *implicit learning*, which is the tendency for people to acquire complex, abstract concepts after being exposed to multiple examples of the patterns. The person learns the pattern through becoming increasingly sensitized to the regularities behind the patterns. Using strings of alphabetic letters (e.g., PVV, TSSSXXVV, TSXXTVPS, etc.) to form an artificial grammar, subjects in Reber's experiments are to judge whether or not each letter set fits the grammar and amazingly they make correct responses about 77% of the time. Implicit learning is a "primitive but powerful form of adaptation." Reber noted that, in this kind of learning, people don't actually search for rules or receive explicit instruction in the rules but are simply exposed to properly formed letter strings. Subjects learn the grammar "the way we learn to speak our native tongue." Brown (2007) explained that, in implicit teaching, the objective is not obviously expressed but is passively suggested or implied. Implicit learning is a passive process happening when a student acquires knowledge simply through exposure to information. It occurs "without intention to learn and without awareness of what has been learned" (Brown, 2007, p. 291). Students are never taught the actual rules during implicit learning but they deduce their own form based on examples provided. Brown offered the following purposes of implicit teaching:

- Introduces new concepts in a student-centered manner;
- Gives students instruction with a variety of several examples, without teaching students the actual grammar rules;
- Allows students to create their own schemas for understanding rules instead of memorizing specific rules, which enables long-term memory retention.

Included among some constraints of this method are:

- Can be difficult for learners to deduce rules
- Vague, unstructured
- Students may misinterpret rules

In *explicit learning*, which is active and intentional, students seek out the structure of information provided them through direct attention being called toward specific objectives in an environment that is highly structured. According to Brown, explicit teaching, which is very teacher-centered, involves modeling thinking patterns. "This involves a teacher thinking out loud while working through a 'problem' to help students understand how they should think about accomplishing a task" (see LanguageLinks, 2006). The purposes of explicit teaching include:

- Introduces a new topic or skill;
- Provides guided instruction for understanding rules, skills, and thinking;
- Gives students specific instruction through modeling, which allows students to develop understanding through practice.

Brown cautioned that, although explicit teaching is effective for logical, mathematics, linguistic, or verbal intelligences and offers straightforward rules, some constraints include:

- Does not offer communicative learning;
- Students memorize rules; it does not enable individualized understanding;
- Generally does not allow for authentic, contextualized learning.

Although there are pros and cons for both implicit and explicit teaching, many researchers have found that a combination of implicit and explicit learning may yield the best results. When I am implicitly introducing a new concept, I will either use multiple examples in play or while I'm drawing or engaging in other activities during the session. Books lend themselves beautifully to the introduction of concepts, utilizing an implicit technique at first and then moving to an explicit format and back again. So, for instance, I might introduce my learner to pronouns using a book with many instances of "he" and "she" and simply read the book two or three times on various occasions to the child. I would point out, from time to time, that "this word says 'she,'" and "this word says 'he.'" As I move toward more explicit teaching, I say "this word says 'she.'"

"What does this word say?" (point to the word "she." Moving more toward explicit teaching, I ask more and more times, "What does this word say?" I might then have the words "she" and "he" printed onto Post-It notes and point to the words and say "This says 'she'" "What does this say?" If the student has begun to read, we will follow this with another book with the words "she" and "he" and I can apply the same implicit model of teaching as I did previously. I move toward explicit teaching when I say "this says 'she,' because we're talking about this girl, Molly" (for instance). "This says 'he,' because we're talking about this boy, Jason" (for instance). In checking for understanding, I have the child read the sentence about Molly and I ask "Why did you say 'she?'" (because it's about Molly). And with the sentence about Jason I say "Why did you say 'he?'" (because it's about Jason).

Why Do Clients Need to Work on These Goals?

From formal or informal testing or other's reported scores and description of the client's needs, the clinician formulates a written plan stating what the client needs to improve. A skeleton of what clinical objectives might look like follows:

> (Client name) will increase/decrease (what behavior) in response to (what input) by (doing what) in (what environment) with (some measurement) usually percent accuracy, number of times in a certain time frame, or how many seconds/minutes does a behavior need to be observed to be considered improved.

A few examples are included here to illustrate.

- Addie will demonstrate increased play skills through engaging in increasingly complex play in response to props in the therapy room over 20 minutes of play.
- Jake will increase receptive language skills by demonstrating understanding of prepositional concepts in response to verbal prompts given by the clinician in the therapy room with 80% accuracy.
- Robbie will increase expressive language skills through combining noun plus verb phrases ("the boy is walking") in response to

visual cues and verbal prompts given by the clinician in the therapy room with 80% accuracy.

The reader is referred to the sources cited earlier by Nelson (1990), and Wilson et al. (2005) for a myriad of suggested goals to be written for children in language therapy.

It is obvious that increased receptive skills lead to better understanding of our language and that increased expressive skills lead to a child's ability to communicate verbally with others more effectively. The question I frequently ask my child language student clinicians is: "Where will your client need to use his/her skills most?" In most cases, the answer is "in school" or "in the classroom." That is where most of our clients will need to perform, to demonstrate increasing oral-written literacy skills. So, rather than working in a vacuum, we must be ever vigilant to tie what we do to what the child needs to perform effectively in his or her classroom. We must tie what we do to the client's curriculum as much as possible. To that end, it is critical that SLPs with school-age clients address how the client will be able to succeed in accessing the curriculum as the result of the goals worked on during language therapy. This work has been done for us in most states through Departments of Education. Although there is wide variation in how states have written their Language Arts Curriculum standards or benchmarks and in how each school district adapts these for their schools, we must tie our clinical goals and objectives to these standards and benchmarks.

The following sample standards and benchmarks are included in the California Language Arts Curriculum for first grade reading and are presented here to illustrate the above discussion.

1.2.0 Reading Comprehension
Comprehension and Analysis of Grade-Level-Appropriate Text

1.2.2 Respond to who, what, when, where, and how questions.
By (annual IEP date), (name) will answer *who, what, when, where, and how* questions from curriculum-relevant texts in classroom tasks, as measured by (objective, rubric, SLS observation, teacher checklist/monitor chart).

■ *By (date of marking period), (name) will answer who, what, where and when questions from a curriculum-*

relevant text read aloud, as measured by (objective, rubric, SLS observation, teacher checklist/monitor chart).

1.2.3 Follow one-step written instructions independently.

By (annual IEP date), (name) will follow one-step written instructions in classroom tasks by demonstrating an understanding of the "instruction words" (i.e., underline, fill in the blank, copy, draw of picture of list, fill in the word, etc) used in curriculum-relevant materials as measured by (objective, rubric, SLS observation, teacher checklist/monitor chart).

■ *By (date of marking period), (name) will identify "instruction words" in classroom curriculum materials as measured by (objective, rubric, SLS observation, teacher checklist/monitor chart).*

1.2.4 Use context to resolve ambiguities about word and sentence meanings.

By (annual IEP date), (name) will clarify misunderstandings about word and sentence meanings (ambiguities) in curriculum-relevant text as measured by (objective, rubric, SLS observation, teacher checklist/monitor chart).

■ *By (date of marking period), (name) will indicate when a misunderstanding about the meaning of a word or sentence is encountered as measured by (objective, rubric, SLS observation, teacher checklist/monitor chart).*

1.2.5 Confirm predictions about what will happen next in text by identifying key words (i.e., signpost words).

By (annual IEP date), (name) will predict and confirm the sequence of events by identifying key words (signpost words) in an curriculum-relevant text as measured by(objective, rubric, SLS observation, teacher checklist/monitor chart).

■ *By (date of marking period), (name) will identify signpost words (i.e., first, next, last, however, then, etc) from curriculum relevant texts as measured by (objective, rubric, SLS observation, teacher checklist/monitor chart).*

1.2.6 Relate prior knowledge to textual information.

By (annual IEP date), (name) will relate prior knowledge to information from curriculum-relevant text/stories as measured by (objective, rubric, SLS observation, teacher checklist/ monitor chart).

■ *By (date of marking period), (name) will respond to clinician prompting about prior knowledge of a topic about curriculum relevant text/stories as measured by (objective, rubric, SLS observation, teacher checklist/monitor chart).*

1.2.7 **Retell the central ideas of simple expository or narrative passages.**

By (annual IEP date), (name) will retell the central ideas of curriculum-relevant passages or stories as measured by (objective, rubric, SLS observation, teacher checklist/monitor chart).

■ *By (date of marking period), (name) will complete a simple graphic organizer including the central ideas of curriculum-relevant passages or stories as measured by (objective, rubric, SLS observation, teacher checklist/ monitor chart).*

Your job, as a speech-language specialist working with school-age children, is to tie your goals and objectives into your state language arts curriculum standards. For example, if your clinical goal is "to increase a client's expressive language through verbally answering questions," you can easily relate this to a goal the student must meet in the classroom such as the California Language Arts first grade Goal 1.2.2: to respond to who, what, when, where and how questions, which was listed above.

Another example: if your clinical goal is "to increase a client's expressive language through increased oral narrative ability," you can tie this to a goal the student must meet in the classroom such as the California Language Arts first grade Goal 1.2.7: to retell the central ideas of simple expository or narrative passages, which was listed above.

What Materials Should Be Used?

As mentioned in the preceding section, you select your goals following your formal and informal testing and the testing results that have come to you from other sources. Then you write your language goals, integrating them into curriculum-based goals, when possible. Next, it is time to select which materials to use. See Chapter 2 for a discussion of what to use during sessions to increase *play* skills.

I gravitated to the use of children's books years go. I found that, when children are becoming tired of "just play," they gravitate toward sitting at a table and begin to prefer books and writing materials. It's as though they "shed their need for play" as they begin searching for more patterns—this time in expressive language skills. For years I used published decks of pictured items and I still use these materials when I need some "drill and kill" materials. By this I mean, when I want to explicitly drill a child on some form such as "irregular past tense," I find it helpful to use picture cards depicting a boy throwing/catching contrasted with the ball that he threw or caught. But picture cards are decontextualized materials. The reason they have been grouped together is because they represent a common theme, in this case, representing present and irregular past tense. We have decks of cards and lists of words in books that represent various categories such as foods, clothes, transportation items, occupations, and so forth. We have similar pictures and lists for working on adjectives, possessives, nouns, and so on. We have them for figurative language including, for instance, metaphors and similes. And these are all good sources for practitioners. But these picture cards and book lists are not related to anything. There is no story into which they have been embedded. They are not grounded in anything; they merely represent some concept or word part, and we ask our client to name the picture or repeat it after we say it and we expect the client to learn the word but what good is this "word" without the client's knowledge of when to use it in his or her world, that is, outside our therapy rooms without those particular pictures or word lists.

Slowly, I moved away from these materials toward those that are contextualized. I think I simply became bored with decontextualized materials in the form of card decks of pictures and lists of words. Contextualized learning "is based on the proposition that people learn more effectively when they are learning about something that they are interested in, that they already know something about, and that affords them the opportunity to use what they already know to figure out new things" (Nwakeze & Seiler, 1993, pp. 17–18). Contextualized materials are brought together around a theme, topic, story, and so forth. The stimulus words are tied to these and used a number of times throughout the material. Children's literature has always fascinated and delighted me and I grew into using children's books more and more in my own therapy. Children's literature provides material in which children can learn many elements of their language while delighting over surprises in events described and colorful words used in descriptions. Many authors have commented on how this medium allows for great imagery (the big bad wolf fell into a tub of hot water) or (Humpty Dumpty fell off a tall brick wall). Contextualized materials provide a rich source for children and adults to learn new vocabulary and language skills in the way in the various ways in which words are put together in our language. Anderson (2006) included the following as a few of the specific benefits children derive from reading and listening to books:

- Strengthening a bond between the child and adult reader
- Experiencing the pleasure of escaping into a fantasy world or an exciting adventure
- Developing a favorable attitude toward books as an enrichment to their lives
- Stimulating cognitive development
- Gaining new vocabulary and syntax
- Becoming familiar with story and text structures
- Stimulating and expanding their imaginations
- Stretching attention spans
- Empathizing with other people's feelings and problems
- Learning ways to cope with their own feelings and problems
- Widening horizons as they vicariously learn about the world
- Developing an interest in new subjects and hobbies
- Understanding the heritage of their own and other cultures (p. 2)

I'll revisit the importance of using contextualized materials in Chapter 5. For purposes of illustration, let's imagine your client's testing revealed a need to increase the correct production of pronouns "he/she" (this seems like it is an almost universal item on some child language tests). You could use any of a number of published picture cards showing girls and women versus boys and men running, driving, jumping, and so on. The "drill and kill" approach is to show your client one picture card after another asking, "Who is walking," model the answer, and expect the answer "she" or "he." How many times have I witnessed my student clinicians targeting he/she pronouns by bringing a girl doll and a boy doll into the therapy room. They spend session after session asking, "Who is _____' (falling, climbing, crying, etc) expecting the answer "he or she is."

Rather than use cards with "he" and "she" pictures, why not read *Blueberries for Sal* (McCloskey, 1948) to your client? Here are a few sample sentences with key pronoun words capitalized here to emphasize their inclusion in the McCloskey book.

> Little Sal brought along HER small tin pail and HER mother brought HER large tin pail to put berries in. We will take our berries home and can them" said HER mother. "Then we will have food for the winter." Little Sal picked three berries and dropped them in HER little tin pail . . . SHE picked three more berries and ate them. Then SHE picked more berries and dropped one in the pail . . . and the rest SHE ate. Then Little Sal ate all four blueberries out of HER pail. Little Sal hurried ahead and dropped a blueberry in HER mother's pail . . . SHE reached down inside to her HER berry back. . . .

> On the other side of Blueberry Hill, Little Bear came with HIS mother to eat blueberries. Little Bear followed behind HIS mother as SHE walked slowly through the bushes eating berries. Little Bear stopped now and then to eat berries. Then HE had to hustle along to catch up. Because HIS feet were tired of hustling, HE picked out a large clump of bushes and sat down right in the middle and ate blueberries . . . By this time, Little Bear had eaten all the berries HE could reach without moving from HIS clump of bushes

And so it goes, using other books on your shelf or listed under pronouns in Gebers' *Books Are for Talking Too!*, 3rd edition (2003), you can find many other sources that include pronouns. Another example of "pronoun rich text" is Freeman's (1976) *Corduroy*. A sample for this text follows:

"Shall I put HIM in a box for YOU?" the saleslady asked. "Oh no thank you," Lisa answered. And SHE carried Corduroy home in HER arms. SHE ran all the way up four flights of stairs, into HER family's apartment, and straight to Her own room. Corduroy blinked. There was a chair and a chest of drawers, and alongside a girl-size bed stood a little bed just the right size for HIM . . . " this must be home," HE said. "I know I'VE always wanted a home!" Lisa sat down with Corduroy on HER lap and began to sew a button on HIS overalls. I like YOU the way YOU are," SHE said,"But YOU'LL be more comfortable with YOUR shoulder strap fastened."

A great example of a book that could be used to introduce a client to prepositional phrases is *There's An Alligator Under My Bed* (Mayer, 1987) A sample of text follows:

There used to be an alligator UNDER MY BED. I put a peanut butter sandwich, some fruit, and the last piece of pie IN THE GARAGE. I put cookies DOWN the hall. I put a soda and some candy NEXT TO MY BED. Then I hid IN THE HALL CLOSET. I followed him DOWN THE STAIRS.

These three examples were included here to illustrate the rich language that exists in children's literature and to underscore my plea to use contextualized materials to implicitly and explicitly teach many of the target goals you included in your children's language intervention program.

The purpose of this chapter was to review some basic rationale for working on early oral-written language skills. To this end, the following topics were covered:

■ Where do goals come from in child language therapy?
■ What are some guiding principles in therapy? This section focused on" the linguistic innateness theory; the theory of neurolinguistic development; humans as pattern seekers and the concept of goodness of fit; and implicit and explicit teaching.

- Why do clients need to work on these goals?
- What materials should be used?

Chapter 5 looks at how to link the strands of language and literacy through practical suggestions on how to facilitate oral-written abilities in children's language.

Remember: Your client may need to have *oral-written language skills* targeted as the first strand to include in his or her language therapy. He or she may demonstrate the need to return to the earlier *play* strand, or he or she may need to revisit the *listening skills* strand while working on later strands.

Chapter 5

Linking the Strands of Oral-Written Language: The How-Tos

*I*nitial strands of language and literacy covered in earlier chapters included: play, listening skills, and the rationale for linking the strands of oral-written language. This chapter describes the "how-tos" of linking the oral and written strands of language and literacy.

Traditionally, definitions of literacy have referred to mastery of written language, including reading and writing. The concept of emergent literacy includes the developmental and interactive relationship between spoken and written language forms. Kaderavek and Justice (2002) explained that *emergent literacy* refers to "children's use and understanding of literacy (and that it) precedes their development of conventional reading and writing abilities" (p. 396). Cabell, Justice, Kaderavik, Turnbull, and Breit-Smith (2009) cautioned:

> It is important not to confuse emergent literacy with early literacy or beginning reading. Children in the emergent stage of development are not beginning readers; they are emergent readers. As emergent "readers," children are not decoding words. Rather, they are reading logographically, as they identify environmental print based on visual cues (e.g., stop sign says "stop"; golden arches for McDonald's). (p. 3)

Justice (2007) explained that the best predictors of decoding and three high priority targets include: phonological awareness, print knowledge, and emergent writing. Nelson (2010) explained that "assessing emergent literacy at the sentence/discourse level should include:

■ Observation of the interest and attention children show when adults try to engage them in interactions with books

- Observations of children listening to books being read aloud
- Observation of signs of children's knowledge about how to hold a book, turn the pages, look at the pictures, point to objects named, point to words (contrasted with pictures), and close and put the book aside when finished. (p. 266)

In her discussion of the importance of emergent literacy, Paul (2007) suggested:

> In working with clients who are functioning in the emerging language stage, we want to emphasize to parents the importance of book reading and storytelling and remind them that their child can benefit from such opportunities. Books chosen for these clients should contain simple pictures that can be labeled or described with a few words . . . showing children simple, attractive pictures in books and labeling them with one- and two-word descriptions will be appropriate for now. (p. 311)

The National Early Literacy Panel (2004) recommendations, as cited by Cabell et al. (2009), identified key emergent literacy skills that are the best predictors of later reading and spelling achievement:

- Oral language including vocabulary and inferential language
- Phonological awareness
- Print awareness
- Alphabet knowledge
- Emergent writing

These headings have been used for the next five sections of this chapter. Under oral language, I have included a section on developing oral-narrative abilities. I added two final sections: Early Reading and Writing, and Problem-Solving/Creative Activities. Each main section includes a description of the topic and suggestions for working on it.

Oral Language

According to Cabell et al. (2009), the oral language component of key emergent literacy skills includes vocabulary and inferential language. I have added a third to this list, oral-narrative language. Cabell et al. (2009) explained that "children's ability to effectively use and comprehend language is an essential precursor to reading. Children who do not develop adequate oral language skills tend to lag behind their peers in literacy" (p. 6). The importance of assessing and teaching various aspects of oral language to facilitate comprehension and production of higher order language and metalinguistic skills proposed by ASHA (2001) included the following:

- Figurative-language forms: sophisticated nonliteral language uses such as idioms, metaphors, proverbs, humor, and poetic language
- Literate lexicon: rarer and more abstract vocabulary that occurs in scholarly contexts
- Synonyms and antonyms: word equivalents and word opposites
- Inferential comprehension and reasoning: the integration of meaning within text, analogies, and verbal problem solving
- Syntactic complexity: clause density, and linguistic cohesion
- Polysemous vocabulary: words that have multiple meanings. (p. 13)

In Chapter 2, suggestions were provided for increasing children's early words and increasing mean length of utterance (MLU) through indirect and direct methods. Many of ASHA's recommendations go beyond the scope of this book, but vocabulary and inferential language skills will be included followed by a section on developing oral narrative skills.

Increasing Vocabulary

According to the National Reading Panel (2000), vocabulary knowledge is critical to the development of reading skills. The panel differentiated types of vocabulary: oral vocabulary and print vocabulary:

> A reader who encounters a strange word in print can decode the word to speech. If it is in the reader's oral vocabulary, the reader will be able to understand it. If the word is not in the reader's oral vocabulary, the reader will have to determine the meaning by other means . . . the larger the reader's vocabulary (either oral or print), the easier it is to make sense of the text. (p. 1)

The NRP noted that "oral vocabulary is a key to learning to make the transition from oral to written forms, whereas reading vocabulary is crucial to the comprehension processes of a skilled reader" (p. 15). Johnson and Yeates (2006) concluded that vocabulary growth occurs at "an astonishing rate throughout childhood" (p. 2.) These authors summarized other's works in documenting vocabulary growth:

- Children learn nine new words daily in preschool years (Carey, 1978)
- Children learn more than 20 words daily during early school years (Anglin, 1993)
- Young children probably acquire most of their new words implicitly by hearing them used in verbal contexts (Hart & Risley, 1995)
- Older children implicitly learn more new words through independent reading (Nagy & Anderson, 1984).

Inferential Knowledge

As children acquire vocabulary, they move from concrete/literal meanings to more inferential language. Pointing out that interactions with preschool-age children "focus on literal language (What color is this? What is Sally doing?)," Cabell et al. (2009) explained that building inferential language is critical to later reading comprehension. "Inferencing skills can be developed in preschoolers long before they begin to read. Inferential language includes language to problem solve and reason as well as discuss cause and effect" (p. 6). Examples might include, "What do you think would happen if Goldilocks had not fallen asleep?" or "What do you think happens next?"

Suggestions for Working on Oral Language

Suggestions for increasing oral language with young children through play were given in Chapter 2. More directive approaches can be found in a number of sources including McCauley and Fey (2006) and Paul (2007). Fey (1986) is credited with describing a continuum of naturalness in language intervention with children. Child-centered approaches such as facilitative play and the Hanen approach mentioned in Chapter 2 are considered to be the most natural in that the adult follows the child's lead and comments on what the child is doing. These techniques are intended to stimulate and support general communication. Less natural approaches known as "hybrid" (described below) include milieu teaching, focused stimulation, and script therapy. Finally, the least natural approach to child language intervention is clinician-directed techniques including drill, drill play, and modeling.

Hybrid Approaches

Hybrid approaches include language stimulation techniques where the "clinician maintains a good deal of control in selecting activities and materials but does so in a way that consciously tempts the child to make spontaneous use of utterances of the types being targeted (Paul, 2007, p. 79).

In *milieu teaching*, the intent is to increase the child's motor or verbal responses. In trying to increase the child's understanding that the adult is a necessary element in the environment to give the child something he or she wants, the environment is set up so that the child will need to engage the adult visually, gesturally, and/or verbally. Objects or toys are placed out of the child's reach or in plastic containers or bags. The child must look at, reach for, vocalize, say a word for the adult to "move in" and get/give the desired item. I encourage student clinicians to "dummy up" here (i.e., don't automatically give something to the child). Greenspan's Floortime approach talks about "playful obstruction" and that would fit here as well. Once the child is interacting with an object, the adult somehow blocks the entrance to something, for instance, leans on the top of the toy box so the child cannot open it without looking at or vocalizing something to the adult. Have your back against a shelf with toys on it. Sit on the floor and block the cupboard with toys in it. It is appropriate for the clinician to look puzzled and ask the child "What?" "What do you want?" "Which car do you want?" As mentioned in Chapter 2, some clinicians occasionally become more directive saying "Use your words;" "Tell me what you want."

In *focused stimulation*, the clinician sets up the interaction so that she or he can provide many examples of a particular verbal form. Similar to auditory bombardment in phonological processes therapy, the adult "bombards" the child with multiple examples of the word or syntactic form targeted. So, for instance, the clinician may comment on the *red* car going through a *red* stoplight, with a policeman with a *red* blinking light on his or her car. It is appropriate for the clinician to provide opportunities for the child to verbalize the targeted word, for instance, "there are lots of red things here—there's the car and the stoplight, and what else?" The child does not have to verbally produce the answer but is given the opportunity to do so. *Vertical structuring* can be used in this approach to expand on what the child has said. For example, the child might say "red" to indicate the red car and the adult can expand this with "yes it is a red car, and it is going fast." Again, the child does not have to repeat the adult's verbalization. As Paul (2007) explained, "The fact that children often imitate adult expansions of their own utterances in normal development is the basis for the hope that children with language impairments will take these expanded models of their own intended utterances as a cue for spontaneous imitation" (pp. 79–80).

Script therapy involves re-enacting a familiar scene the child has encountered such as going to the doctor, playing at the park, cooking dinner, or going to a favorite restaurant. The same play materials and script are used over and over and the adult gradually adds to and changes the script. The familiarity of the script is comfortable and the child can be expected to verbalize increasingly longer utterances during the play scene. New words can be added or variations made to what is happening as the child "owns" more of the script. With one of my young clients, cooking dinner with mom and dad was very important. She chose to re-enact going to the store with dad to buy eggs and then coming home and scrambling them with him. The script went something like this: Dad: "kids, I'm going to the store for eggs. Come on." At the store, my client said: "Dad, where are the eggs?" Dad said: "Over here." Back home Dad said: "Kids, get the spoon. Let's stir." And so on. Each session we re-enacted this and gradually added to the play scenario with serving the eggs, eating the eggs, and cleaning up afterward. The script became increasingly complex, for instance, dad asked the kids to "get into the car. We're going to buy eggs at the store. The grocery store." And at the store the script became: "Kids, the white eggs are over here. I'm at the egg aisle. Come find me. Let's buy these white eggs." I have found that children love this approach and will build on the script until the scenario becomes "old" to them, and then it's time to move to a new script. Start with descriptions of the basic events and gradually add to the script/scenario.

There is no rule here. Children will let you know if they like what you add in. If they don't like something you will hear a resounding "no" or "He didn't say that!"

Clinician-Directed Approaches

Paul (2007) explained that with clinician-directed techniques in child language therapy, the "clinician specifies materials to be used, how the client will use them, the type and frequency of reinforcement, the form of the responses to be accepted as correct, and the order of activities—in short, all aspects of the intervention . . . and have proven efficacy in eliciting new language forms" (pp. 74–75). These approaches include drill, drill play, and modeling.

Drill activities involve the clinician telling the child what she or he should say; perhaps using a motivating event; prompting the child as to what the child should say, which can be faded, and reinforcement. For example, the clinician may set up a racetrack with cars racing across the table or floor and the child is told to say "Stop" so the cars won't crash. A prompt might be "use your word," or "say /st/." The reinforcement in this case might be giving the car to the child to race.

Drill play is similar to a drill activity with the addition of another motivating event. Using the above example of race cars, the child may now be allowed to choose the race car that needs to stop, race it, say "Stop," and finish racing that car.

In *modeling* the clinician or another child or adult models, verbally producing the word(s) similar to focused stimulation described above. The difference in modeling is that the child is not immediately required to verbalize the utterance(s) but just to listen. Once again, there is similarity to the auditory bombardment approach used to improve phonological processes. The clinician or other person in the room produces 10 to 20 examples of the target word or syntactic form. Then the child is asked to describe another set of objects or pictured items. For instance, if the descriptor number "2" is targeted, the clinician or other person can name "two cars," "two birds," "two apples," and so on, and then the child is shown additional pairs of objects and asked to "talk like" the adult did so perhaps saying "two keys," "two crayons," and so forth.

I typically use a combination of the above approaches when working with young children who are increasing verbalizations, and when they are beginning to expand utterances. Because of my deep conviction that vocabulary isn't learned easily from decontextualized materials, I frequently use books to teach new words (see later topics in this chapter). You can select books based on what vocabulary or concepts you want to teach. If you want to use books to teach specific vocabulary more directly, I recommend Jane O'Connor's books about Fancy Nancy. *In Fancy Nancy and the Posh Puppy* (O'Connor, 2007), Nancy says "Then I get an idea that is spectacular. (That's a fancy word for great.) And she says "My dad says Frenchy is a LaSalle spaniel. That is a very unique breed. (Unique is fancy for one of a kind). The Lemony Snicket books provide a similar approach to expanding vocabulary for older students. Some specific goals for increasing concepts and vocabulary include but are not limited to:

- Increase vocabulary to include: antonyms and synonyms; word-finding activities; identifying word meanings; labeling; and defining words
- Increase understanding and use of language concepts including but not limited to sequencing events; categories (naming the superordinate category as well as subordinate category members); similarities and differences; analogies; always/never/sometimes; and idioms
- Increase understanding and use of routinized sequences such as days of the week, months of the year, the seasons, and so forth.
- Increase use of propositions (combining thoughts) with words such as "and," "next," "because" through play and educational games such as, "What's in a Square."

Qualitative Analysis of Test Items

Now it's time to return to the test manual(s) you used during assessment to do an item analysis and to investigate what lies behind items included in a particular test. This allows for a qualitative analysis of test items, designed to lead more directly to what a particular child needs to have included in his or her remedial program at this point to increase oral language. To illustrate this, I have chosen some subtests from frequently used child language tests.

Clinical Evaluation of Language Fundamentals (CELF-4) (Semel et al., 2003)

Subtest: Concepts and Following Directions

According to the test manual, this subtest "evaluates the student's ability to (a) interpret spoken directions of increasing length and complexity, containing concepts that require logical operations; (b) remember the names, characteristics, and order of mention of objects; and (c) identify from among several choices the pictured objects that were mentioned" (p. 19). Included in the item analysis of the subtest are the following concepts:

Inclusion/Exclusion: all/except; all, all but; all but one; neither/nor; and

Location: top, next to, farthest, closest to, between, top/bottom, separated, right/ left

Sequence: beginning, last, first, middle, second, fourth, third

Condition: unless

Temporal: after, before, same time, while, then

If a child scores poorly on this subtest, it shows a weakness in his or her ability to follow directions for lessons, assignments, and activities, both in the classroom and in the home.

Suggested Goals

1. Increase ability to follow auditory directions
2. Increase knowledge of relational concepts

Suggested Therapy Activities. Integrate simple (one-step) activities in sessions and build up child's skill level by increasing complexity. You may want to begin with helping the child motor through activities, and then decreasing cuing over time. Introduce relational concepts including prepositions (e.g., over, under, next to), superlatives (e.g., far, farther, farthest), descriptive and dimensional terms (e.g., big/little, red/yellow).

Materials Might Include

- Simple verbal command games: Mother May-I; Red-light/ green light; Head-Shoulders-Knees and Toes; Hokey Pokey
- Simple craft activities requiring sequencing of steps (including activities that involve color, size, shape, differences in materials)

Subtest: Word Structure

According to the test manual, this subtest "evaluates the student's ability to (a) apply word structure rules (morphology) to mark inflections, derivations, and comparison; and (b) select and use appropriate pronouns to refer to people, objects, and possessive relationships" (p. 23).

Included among the item analysis of the subtest are the following:

Regular Plural: books, horses

Irregular Plural: mice, children

Third Person Singular: reads, flies

Possessive Nouns: Paula's boot, king's/queen's

Derivation of Nouns: singer

Contractible Copula: She is/She's happy

Auxiliary + -ing: is listening; is eating; are swinging/jumping

Possessive Pronouns: yours

Regular Past Tense: climbed

If a child scores poorly on this subtest, it shows a weakness in his or her linguistic flexibility; it reflects a weakness in the use of a variety of word structures: morphology, pronouns, nouns, inferences to time and numbers, possessive relationships, and comparisons.

Suggested Goals

1. Increase use of morphological endings
2. Increase knowledge of time and number inferences
3. Increase expressive language abilities

Suggested Therapy Activities. Integrate word structures into play activities, such as daily events (cooking, playing house, playing doctor, race cars), or charade-like games that encourage the child to use the missing (or weak) word forms, for example, if a game card says running, the child acts out that action and then labels the action in discussion: "*I am running.*"

Materials Might Include

Imaginary play toys: tea set, action figures/dolls, play set (cooking, house, tool sets) to elicit target word forms

Simple craft activities with discussions of actions during the activities, numbers of items used to make object, comparisons between materials (big/little, under/on)

Simple verbal command games: Mother May-I; Red-light/green light; Head-Shoulders-Knees and Toes; Hokey Pokey

Simple craft activities requiring sequencing of steps (including activities that involve color, size, shape, differences in materials)

Test of Narrative Development (TNL) (Gillam & Pearson, 2004)

The TNL "measures children's ability to answer questions about stories, to retell stories and to create their own stories. To perform these tasks, children must formulate interrelated ideas about characters, their goals, their actions, and the outcomes of those actions. Then, they must weave strings of words, phrases, and sentences together in ways that represent sequential and causal relationships between the characters, actions, and outcomes" (p. vii.).

Included in the item analysis of the subtests are the following concepts:

Events: temporal relationships between events (e.g., "and" "then"; adverbial phrases "after" "as he was")

Grammar: causal relationships: because, since, so, therefore

Story: tell how each statement (subject-verb-object unit) relates to the story as a whole; story is complete, creative/well organized; setting; characters; indicates a problems or conflict; actions/events; indicates causal relationships between actions/events; consequences or resolution, and provides an ending

Suggested Goals

1. Increase use of adverbial phrase usage: after/before
2. Increase use of causal relationship words: because, since, so therefore
3. Increase story-telling skills
4. Maintain verb tense while telling a story
5. Using oral narrative outlines/story boards (see accompanying CD) tell a story including setting, events, character(s), problem/conflict, actions/events, consequences, ending, how the character felt.

Suggested Therapy Activities. See next section on Oral Narrative Skills

Materials Might Include. See accompanying CD

Increasing Oral Narrative Skills

According to Nelson (2010) "narratives organize experience into interpretable wholes that are more than just a series of connected sentences. They present opportunities for facilitating more complex language comprehension and production and for engaging young children in literate language experiences as well" (p. 308). Using a standard story-retelling task in 4-year-olds with language disabilities, Bishop and Edmundson (1987) found narrative skill was one of the best predictors of later school success. Paul and Smith (1993) explained that a number of higher level language and cognitive skills are involved in the ability to tell a story. These include:

- the ability to sequence events
- to create a cohesive text through the use of explicit linguistic markers
- to use precise vocabulary
- to convey ideas without extralinguistic support

■ to understand cause-effect relationships
■ and to structure the narration along the lines of universal story schemata that aid the listener in comprehending the tale. (p. 592)

Owens (2010) explained that "oral narration includes the telling of self-generated stories, storytelling of familiar tales, retelling of movies or television shows, and recounting of personal experiences. Most conversations include narratives of this latter type" (p. 217). Owens cited a number of researchers' findings that illuminate some of the characteristics of oral narrative abilities in children with language disorders compared with typically developing children. Some of these include:

■ narratives are shorter and less mature
■ narratives have less mature episode and sentence structure
■ children with language problems convey and recall less information
■ children with language disorders retrieve less information and make fewer inferences
■ children with language issues contain the elements in the generally appropriate order, they are substantially shorter and contain fewer and more poorly organized complete episodes
■ more statements made by children with language problems are not integrated into the episode structure
■ children with language problems exhibit a greater rate of communication breakdown
■ children with language problems use conjunctions but are less efficient in their use
■ children with language problems often fail to consider the needs of their audience
■ children with language problems use less and incomplete internal story organization. (p. 217)

In her master's degree project, Spitler-Kashuba (2009) summarized the narrative, language, and theory of mind developmental milestones as presented by McCabe and Rollins (1992), Norbury and Bishop (2003), Paul (2001), Saracho and Spodek (2006), Westby and McKellar (2000), and Shipley and McAfee (2004). Table 5–1 should prove useful to the practitioner as she or he considers what to include in the client's development of oral narrative skills.

Table 5–1. Narrative, Language and Theory of Mind (ToM) Developmental Milestones

Age	Narrative Skills	Language Skills	ToM Skills
12 mos		• First real words; nouns, familiar people or objects	• Communicates desire with eye contact; joint attention develops • Points to object
18 mos		• Uses up to 100 words • Understands basic what, who, where questions	• Begins to use words to get needs met
22 mos	• Begins to refer to past events with assistance from an adult	• "Telegraphic" utterances • Primarily CVC words, multi-syllable words begin to emerge	• Begins to request information and answer questions
2 yrs	• Personal narratives begin with a focus on negative past events • "Heap stories" including just labels and descriptions	• Uses 50 to 250 words • Begins to combine words • Starts to ask/answer questions • Enjoys listening to stories	• Talks about the absence of objects ("all gone") • May misrepresent reality; lie, tease
3 yrs	• Two events appear in narratives • By 36 mo: "sequences" form, theme but without plan of action • Between 36 to 42 mo: "primitive" narratives emerge —theme and some temporal organization	• Rapid language growth period • Uses 800 words or more • 2- to 4-word phrases • Continues to exhibit multiple grammatical errors	• Maintains topic for several turns

Table 5–1. *continued*

Age	Narrative Skills	Language Skills	ToM Skills
4 yrs	• Begins to create "chain" stories (e.g., . . . and then . . . and then . . .) • Narratives include: some plot and "high point" (conclusion) • Creates imaginary roles with use of props • Uses hints to express desires	• Uses around 1,500 words • Uses conjunctions: so, when, if, because • Understands when and how questions • Understood 100% of the time by an unknown listener	• Predicts behavior or situations • Expresses empathy • Maintains interactions for longer periods
5–6 yrs	• "True" narrative emerges, with a focus on: past personal events, multiple events, and typically ending at story's "high point" • Story grammar elements: "most" use initiating events, 50% include steps taken by characters, 20% share a story conclusion	• Vocabulary continues to increase • Uses 4- to 6-word sentences • Sentences contain details • Generates accurate grammar most of the time	• Understands people can hold false beliefs • Relates experiences in which child felt sad, mad, happy, etc.
6–7 yrs	• Narrative structure is more complete, including central theme/focus, high point and resolution	• Verbal descriptions are more developed • Continues to develop conversational abilities	• Understands "nested" beliefs (e.g., Mommy thinks . . .) • Relates experiences in which the child felt jealous, guilty, etc.

continues

Table 5–1. *continued*

Age	Narrative Skills	Language Skills	ToM Skills
6–7 yrs *continued*		• Constructs sentences approximately 6 words in length • Uses morphological elements accurately most of the time • Understands most concepts of time	
7–9 yrs	• Stories contain greater complexity: character motivations, reactions, and internal goals	• Uses around 5000 words • Pronoun agreement improves • Understanding of multiple meaning words improves	• Continues to develop perspective-taking in order to persuade others
9–14 yrs	• At 9 yrs: still has difficulty formulating story conclusion • 10 yrs: Most story grammar elements are in place, but "higher level language," including pronoun agreements, are still not completely mastered • By 12 yrs: stories include greater episodic complexity (e.g., interactive, embedded episodes)	• Understanding of figurative language continues to improve • Students are expected to acquire new information through reading (including expository texts) • Vocabulary from school texts becomes more abstract • Metacognitive skills emerge	• Understands jokes based on lexical ambiguity, then later based on deep structural ambiguity

One of the reasons I included oral narration under oral language development is to emphasize the importance of including it in language therapy goals and its ties to the current State Language Arts Curriculum Standards. I have included a few relevant ones from California's standards for first grade in the areas of Speaking, Reading, and Writing.

1.2.0 Speaking Application (Genres and Their Characteristics)

1.2.2 Retell stories using basic story grammar, sequencing story events by answering who, what, when, where, why, and how questions.

By (annual IEP date), (name) will retell stories in correct sequence by answering who, what, when, where, why and how questions in classroom tasks.

- *By (date of marking period), (name) will answer /wh/ questions after hearing a story, when given repetitions and cueing as needed.*
- *By (date of marking period), (name) will retell a story in correct sequence, using a "first, next, last" sequence words, as measured by (objective, rubric, SLS observation, teacher checklist/ monitor chart).*

1.2.3 Relate an important life event or personal experience using simple sequencing.

By (annual IEP date), (name) will relate an important life event or personal experience in sequence using temporal cohesive ties when needed in classroom activities as measured by (objective, rubric, SLS observation, teacher checklist/monitor chart).

- *By (date of marking period), (name) will use appropriate temporal cohesive ties (then, when, before, after) when relating an important life event or personal experience, with visual support, as measured by (objective, rubric, SLS observation, teacher checklist/monitor chart).*
- *By (date of marking period), (name) will use appropriate temporal cohesive ties (then, when, before, after) when relating an important life event or personal experience, without visual support, as measured by (objective, rubric, SLS observation, teacher checklist/monitor chart).*

1.2.0 Reading Comprehension
Comprehension and Analysis of Grade-Level-Appropriate Text

1.2.2 Respond to who, what, when, where, and how questions.

By (annual IEP date), (name) will answer *who, what, when, where, and how* questions from curriculum-relevant texts in classroom tasks, as measured by (objective, rubric, SLS observation, teacher checklist/monitor chart).

■ *By (date of marking period), (name) will answer who, what, where and when questions from a curriculum-relevant text read aloud, as measured by (objective, rubric, SLS observation, teacher checklist/monitor chart).*

■ *By (date of marking period), (name) will answer how questions from a curriculum- relevant text read aloud, as measured by (objective, rubric, SLS observation, teacher checklist/monitor chart).*

1.2.5 Confirm predictions about what will happen next in text by identifying key words (i.e., signpost words).

By (annual IEP date), (name) will predict and confirm the sequence of events by identifying key words (signpost words) in an curriculum-relevant text as measured by (objective, rubric, SLS observation, teacher checklist/monitor chart).

■ *By (date of marking period), (name) will identify signpost words (i.e., first, next, last, however, then, etc) from curriculum relevant texts as measured by (objective, rubric, SLS observation, teacher checklist/monitor chart).*

■ *By (date of marking period), (name) will predict events that could happen next in curriculum-relevant by identifying signpost words as measured by (objective, rubric, SLS observation, teacher checklist/monitor chart).*

1.2.6 Relate prior knowledge to textual information.

By (annual IEP date), (name) will relate prior knowledge to information from curriculum-relevant text/stories as measured by (objective, rubric, SLS observation, teacher checklist/monitor chart).

■ *By (date of marking period), (name) will respond to clinician prompting about prior knowledge of a topic about curriculum relevant text/stories as measured by (objective, rubric, SLS observation, teacher checklist/monitor chart).*

■ *By (date of marking period), (name) will relate prior knowledge about given topics from curriculum-relevant text/stories, with minimal prompting by clinician, as measured by (objective, rubric, SLS observation, teacher checklist/monitor chart).*

1.2.7 Retell the central ideas of simple expository or narrative passages.

By (annual IEP date), (name) will retell the central ideas of curriculum-relevant passages or stories as measured by (objective, rubric, SLS observation, teacher checklist/monitor chart).

■ *By (date of marking period)), (name) will complete a simple graphic organizer including the central ideas of curriculum-relevant passages or stories as measured by (objective, rubric, SLS observation, teacher checklist/monitor chart).*

■ *By (date of marking period), (name) will retell the central ideas of curriculum-relevant passages or stories using a completed simple graphic organizer as visual support as measured by (objective, rubric, SLS observation, teacher checklist/monitor chart).*

1.3.0 Literary Response and Analysis
Narrative Analysis of Grade-Level-Appropriate Text

1.3.1 Identify and describe the story elements of plot, setting, and characters, including the story's beginning, middle, and ending.

By (annual IEP date), (name) will identify and describe the story elements of plot, setting and characters, including the story's beginning, middle, and ending, after listening to and/or reading a curriculum-relevant story as measured by (objective, rubric, SLS observation, teacher checklist/monitor chart).

■ *By (date of marking period), (name) will identify beginning, middle and ending of a story (after listening to or reading) using a simple story map as visual support as measured by (objective, rubric, SLS observation, teacher checklist/monitor chart).*

■ *By (date of marking period), (name) will identify theme, plot, setting and characters of a story (after listening to or reading) using a story map as a visual support as measured by (objective, rubric, SLS observation, teacher checklist/monitor chart).*

1.3.3 Recollect, talk, and write about books read during the school year.

By (annual IEP date), (name) will remember, talk and write about books (classroom books, self-selected books and books from curriculum) read during the school year as measured by (objective, rubric, SLS observation, teacher checklist/monitor chart).

■ *By (date of marking period), (name) will recall and talk about selected books/stories using visual supports (graphic organizer, pictures, icons, etc). as measured by (objective, rubric, SLS observation, teacher checklist/monitor chart).*

■ *By (date of marking period), (name) will use visual supports to write about (story frames, graphic organizers) previously-read books/stories as measured by (objective, rubric, SLS observation, teacher checklist/monitor chart).*

1.1.0 Written and Oral English Language Conventions
Sentence Structure

1.1.1 Write and speak in complete, coherent sentences.

By (annual IEP date), when given a verbal or visual cue, (name) will use complete sentences in classroom speaking/writing tasks as measured by (objective, rubric, SLS observation, teacher checklist/monitor chart).

■ *By (date of marking period), when given a verbal or visual cue, (name) will speak in complete sentence of more than words as measured by (objective, rubric, SLS observation, teacher checklist/monitor chart).*

■ *By (date of marking period), when given a*
verbal or visual cue, (name) will write in
complete sentences of at least words as measured
by (objective, rubric, SLS observation, teacher
checklist/monitor chart)

Spitler-Kashuba's (2009) work highlighted the need to work on personal narrative (stories about self) prior to fictional narrative (stories about others). Personal narrative development within the classroom or therapy room may be most successfully accomplished through doing some activity with the child so that you have a shared experience with him or her. Going on a walk, making something during the session, playing a game together are examples of some things that you can do with a child and then "come to the table" to represent the event(s) so the child learns about the importance of retelling what just happened. Take pictures and immediately print them or draw stick figures to represent "what we did first," "next," "then," and "last" to encourage retelling what just occurred. Converting these pictures or drawings into a "book" or journal to send home to parents or caretakers will facilitate carryover practice of oral narrative skills. As personal narratives develop, it is time to move to fictional narratives involving the retell of stories. I prefer using children's literature here to "ground" children in retelling stories read to them to include story aspects such as main character(s), setting, problem, steps to solve the problem, feelings the main character(s) has/have; ending. (See Chaper 6 and accompanying CD.)

I introduce children to books that have very simple story to retell. I might begin with a book as simple as *Where's Spot* (Hill, 1980). I read the book to the child and talk about who the story is about (Spot and his mother), where does the story take place (at home), what is the problem (mom can't find Spot), what happens (Spot's mother finds Spot), and how does Spot's mom feel at the end of the book (happy).

I like to follow this kind of book up with books that include a number of events that happen but not yet needing concepts from oral narrative such as problems, solutions, and feelings. A book such as *Maisy Drives the Bus* (Cousins, 2000) includes Maisy driving her bus and the events include wondering who will be at the various bus stops. Thus, at bus stop number 1, it's Cyril, and Black Cat at bus stop number 2, and Tallulah at stop number 3. This provides children with a sequence of events that doesn't need to be coordinated with anything but bus stop number and the connecting word "next/then." At this point, I almost always add in the hand signs for "first," "next," and "last." I usually then use books with a simplified story such as Cousins' *Maisy Makes Lemonade* (2000), which allows us to add in a problem and solution and how the characters probably feel at the end of the book. In the Lemonade book, Maisy the mouse makes lemonade at home with the help of her friend Eddie the elephant. The problem occurs when Eddie drinks the lemonade. Maisy and Eddie resolve the problem by picking more lemons, squeezing the lemons, adding ice, water, and sugar to the pitcher, which provides us a nice sequence of events. The story ends with Maisy and Eddie drinking lemonade together and we can infer that the characters "feel happy" because they resolved the problem.

In *Maisy's Bedtime* (Cousins, 1999), Maisy the mouse is sleepy and wants to go to bed. The sequence of events that follows includes things that happen in getting ready for bedtime including leaving her stuffed animal, Panda, somewhere. Maisy washes her face, brushes her teeth, puts on pajamas, reads a story and then must find Panda. And in *Maisy Goes Shopping* (Cousins, 2001), Maisy and her crocodile friend, Charley, want to eat lunch. The problem is that Charley's "fridge" is empty. The problem is solved when Maisy and Charley go shopping. They buy apples, bananas, juice, bread, cheese, and yogurt and then return home to eat lunch. These books are perfect to help young children enter into fictional narrative development as they contain the elements needed in a short, delightful story. Carle's *The Secret Birthday Message* (1972) cleverly uses pictured geometric and other shapes to tell a story about a boy named Tim who receives a strange envelope under his pillow on his birthday. On the first page, a half circle is shown above the sentence "When the moon comes up" and a pictured star appears on the second page above the printed sentence "Look for the biggest star." Each page follows with a pictured item including the last page with a pictured rectangle above the printed sentences: "You will see an opening. Climb up and through. That's where you'll find your birthday gift!" A cut-out rectangle appears on the next page where the eyes of a puppy appear.

I gradually move to more complex books including Laura Numeroff's wonderful books. In *If You Give a Mouse a Cookie*

(1985), a hungry mouse gets fed a cookie and will then ask for a glass of milk. He'll look in the mirror to clean his milk mustache and notices a hair and will ask for scissors to cut it. After a series of events the mouse is thirsty and asks for a glass of milk and the story ends with "And chances are if he asks for a glass of milk, he's going to want a cookie to go with it." The Numeroff books include the ingredients for fictional narrative with much more detail and sequence of events than the Cousins books and provide rich extension materials for the ongoing pursuit of oral narrative development. More complex stories can be found in books by Jan Brett. For instance, in *The Mitten: A Ukranian Folktale* (1989), a boy named Nicki wanted new mittens and his grandmother, Baba, knitted a pair for him. Nicki went outside and dropped one of his mittens in the snow. A number of animals including a mole, a snowshoe rabbit, a hedgehog, an owl, a badger, a fox , and so on. find the mitten and go inside for warmth. When the bear sneezes, the mitten is blown into the sky, the animals scatter in all directions, and Nicki regains his mitten. This and other Brett books lend themselves nicely to oral narrative development. The Brett books are filled with beautiful artwork and pages on the left provide a drawing depicting what happened on the last page and the drawing on the right side page previews what will happen next.

For a number of years, I have had my graduate students in Childhood Language Disorders develop their oral narrative outlines (ONOs) around children's books. They select a favorite child's book and develop ONOs that are specific and generic. They can be simplistic or as elaborate as the student wants to be. A simple "specific story strip" can be used with specific pictures from the chosen book to remind the child to retell the story with the elements discussed. The more "generic" story strip removes the pictures specific to the book and only has general, perhaps, stick figures, to help the child retell the fictional narrative. Finally, the child is asked to retell the story from memory without visual aid. The CD that accompanies this book provides extensive examples of fictional narrative using children's literature. Lambert chose to use "story boards" rather than story strips in her materials for oral narrative development.

The following quick reference guide in Table 5–2 was provided by Spitler-Kashuba (2009) to guide us in using a multimodal approach to developing personal and fictional oral narratives.

Table 5–2. A Quick Reference Guide to a Multimodal Approach to Oral Narrative Development

1. GENERAL APPROACHES	2. GET READY TO INTERACT
• Sequential presentation • Repeated exposure to concepts • Conversation & collaboration • Contextualized teaching • Parent/caregiver involvement	• Get on the child's level • Increase your affect • Model language & slow your rate of speech slightly • Don't rush the child

3. EXPAND AND EXPLORE

Personal Narrative	Fictional Narrative

1. Adopt a conversational style
  • Ask open-ended questions
  • Introduce a simple narrative structure (e.g., first, next, last) to help the child organize his thoughts
  • Add greater complexity once the child has mastered this simple structure
2. Follow the child's lead
  • Think collaboration
  • Pause for input
  • Watch & listen
  • Encourage contributions
  • Expand on the child's thought
  • Allow the child to help record their story, when appropriate, through drawings, text or other means.
    – Create books of the child's stories when possible to allow the child to share with others and support emergent literacy skills
3. Model narrative language or "story words" (including the terms: first, next, then, last)
  • See Multimodal Toolbox below for information about teaching story grammar
4. Teach and chart "cause and effect" sequences in stories
	1. Adopt a conversational approach during shared book reading
	  • Relate fictional stories to the child's life through conversation
	2. Follow the child's lead
	  • Think collaboration
	  • Pause for input
	  • Watch & listen
	  • Encourage contributions
	  • Expand on the child's thought
	During shared book reading:
	  • Let the child where to read
	  • Give the child opportunities to hold and manipulate the book
	  • Match the child's interests and abilities—as children age, they become more interested in the story presented by the text, first, talk about pictures
	  • Have the child "read" to you (Justice & Kaderavek, 2002, p. 10)
	3. Model narrative language or "story words" (including the terms: first, next, then, last)
	  • See Multimodal Toolbox below for information about teaching story grammar
	4. Teach and chart "cause and effect" sequences in stories

Table 5–2. *continued*

4. THE MULTIMODAL "TOOLBOX"

Mix and match activities to meet the specific strengths of your child and address narrative language goals

PERSONAL NARRATIVE—Multimodal Activities

Auditory	*Visual*	*Kinesthetic*
Dialogue about daily or past events	**Pictograph events of a child's story**	**Talk about how your body shows emotions**
• Ask for specific information sequences (e.g., Tell me 2 things you had for breakfast? How do you make cereal?).	**&/or**	• Talk about and practice facial expressions and body postures.
	Use symbols to mark story grammar	
	&/or	• Discuss and encourage the use of emotion during storytelling or book reading activities.
• Avoid broad questions that may overwhelm or confuse your child (e.g., What did you do today?).	**Create a "treasure map" or visual time line** to represent the sequence of events.	
Use the "story words" *first, next, then, last* **during story creation and/or retell**	**Use photographs from a child's life** (e.g., family, pets, activities) or take photos of therapy activities to aid story creation.	**Role play story events** as well as character actions and reactions
With younger children, introduce just *first*, *next*, and *last*, including alternative words like *then* only after the others are used consistently.		• First, the adult can review the story pictographs and/or notes, while the child acts out events again.
	Construct "books" of a child's experiences and stories whenever possible	• Next, the adult can act out events while the child "reads" the pictographs.
	ME books, How-to books, social stories or of how to address a child's fears	• With an older child, the adult and child can role-play verbally to explore difficult situations and alternative solutions.
	This scaffolds their narrative language and also supports early literacy skills.	

continues

Table 5–2. *continued*

PERSONAL NARRATIVE—Multimodal Activities *continued*

Auditory	*Visual*	*Kinesthetic*
Teach one story grammar concept at a time, over time* *Character(s)*—who *Setting(s)*—where *Problem*—what (Feelings/Emotions—reactions) *Actions/Steps taken*—how, why *Conclusion*—what (Feelings at the end—reactions) • Teach one concept over several sessions. • Create personal stories to introduce a story grammar concept. • Extend teaching by finding examples of story grammar concept within several storybooks to support learning.	**Encourage a child to take the role of artist** • Teach your child about materials and how they are used. • Encourage critical thinking by discussing composition and art terminology. • Use art to interpret and reflect upon personal stories. • The artistic process can also be a narrative opportunity —help your child chart progress as he or she makes something (via pictographs or drawings) and after the activity is done, sequence steps taken.	**Use sign language or modified sign to mark the "story words" first, next, then, last** • Teach your child hand signs to represent terms. • Model the signs and ask the child to help you remember which word to use when story-telling. • Pause—allow your child to contribute a sign when the time comes. You and your child can practice using story words during shared book reading (e.g., child signs/says "next" for a page to be turned).
Use intonation to retell stories and encourage the child to do the same This helps the child understand and/or think about a story's content, including meaning, emotions and outcomes.	**Transcribe and draw your child's story** **Or, have your child write a simple sentence and produce a simple drawing for each sequence of his story.**	**Encourage dramatic storytelling** • Adults can help anchor ideas or events if they use dramatic body movements while telling stories. It helps your child if you are goofy—get into character!

Table 5–2. *continued*

PERSONAL NARRATIVE—**Multimodal Activities** *continued*

Auditory	*Visual*	*Kinesthetic*
• Younger kids: practice by "picture-walking" through book, looking at illustrations and asking, "What do you think he's saying?" Be dramatic! • Older kids: practice intonation by reading comic strips—the adult can be one character and the child another.	• Remember, children may produce richer language with only pictures as stimuli (no text). • If a child uses pictographs to tell his story, the adult can add text using Post-It notes, if it is appropriate for the child's goals.	• Even if a child does not want to get up and role-play, they can sit and create hand or arm gestures or facial expressions to represent story events and actions.

FICTIONAL NARRATIVE—**Multimodal Activities**

Auditory	*Visual*	*Kinesthetic*
Have conversations about the book you are reading with your child **Discuss ideas in books during shared book reading** • Respond to your child's comments—what in the book is important to them? • Attempt to tie story characters, situations and emotions to the child's life and personal experiences.	**Use story illustrations to improve story comprehension** • Picture walk: when introducing a new story, look through the book with your child. Talk about the illustrations. Ask your child what they think the story is about. • During shared book reading, talk about how pictures can help tell the story and show character qualities and emotions. **Book suggestions:** • Ask your therapist and/or teacher for names of good books for your child.	**Talk about how your body shows emotions** Review the facial expressions and body language of story characters. • Have the child pretend to be a character in a book and do what the book character does. • Review the story emotions in sequence.

continues

Table 5–2. *continued*

FICTIONAL NARRATIVE—Multimodal Activities *continued*

Auditory	*Visual*	*Kinesthetic*
	• Use flip books or books that a child manipulates during reading. • Find books with text that repeats during the book to encourage greater child participation. • Look for books that rhyme or have other sound patterns that support language and literacy development (e.g., alliteration/first words that sound the same).	
Use the "story words" *first, next, then,* **and** *last* **during book reading and/or story retell** • *During shared book reading:* for children who are not fluent readers, use Post-It notes to mark narrative language during book reading (e.g., on the first page, place a Post-It with "First" on it). Simplify the story text or put the story in your own words, as appropriate for your child.	**Use photocopied illustrations to help story retelling** After multiple readings, your child can organize laminated copies of illustrations and retell the story.	**Role play story events as well as character actions and reactions** • The adult can retell or reread the story while the child acts out events. • Then, the adult can act out events while the child "reads" the pictures or text. • With an older child, the adult and child can role-play together and create alternative endings, if appropriate.

Table 5–2. *continued*

Auditory	*Visual*	*Kinesthetic*
• *With story retell:* picture-walk through the book and have your child help you use your "story words" as you talk about each page.		**Play and language:** Imaginative play supports language acquisition and narrative activities. Encourage children to reenact story events using dolls and other toys.
Teach one story grammar concept at a time, over time* **Character(s)**—who **Setting(s)**—where **Problem**—what **(Feelings/Emotions**—reactions) **Actions/Steps taken**—how, why **Conclusion**—what **(Feelings at the end**—reactions) • Teach one concept over several sessions. • Create personal stories to introduce a story grammar concept. • Extend teaching by finding examples of story grammar concept within several storybooks to support learning.	**Encourage a child to take the role of artist** Discuss illustration composition in book read—talk about how to tell a story through pictures. • Teach your child about materials and how they are used. • Encourage critical thinking by discussing composition and art terminology (e.g., shadow, form). • Encourage your child to make a preliminary sketch, and have him make decisions about what to include and exclude in his illustrations. • Discuss materials and mediums—what materials convey the feelings of the story?	**Use sign language or modified sign to mark the "story words"** *first, next, then, last* • Teach your child hand signs to represent terms. • Model the signs and ask your child to make them along with you. • Pause and cue to encourage your child to contribute a sign when the time comes.

continues

129

Table 5–2. *continued*

FICTIONAL NARRATIVE—Multimodal Activities *continued*

Auditory	*Visual*	*Kinesthetic*
	Critique the illustrations in the book you are reading together.	
	• Group work: assign each child a different story event to illustrate.	
Use intonation during the reading and retelling of stories	**Use wordless books to prompt fictional story creation**	**Encourage dramatic storytelling**
This helps the child understand and/or think about a story's content, including meaning, emotions and outcomes.	Look through a wordless book before you share it with your child. This allows you to know the story's events and outcomes.	• Adults can help anchor ideas or events when they use hand and body gestures while telling stories. (This works particularly well when stories include repeating language and/or events.)
• Practice intonation by reading comic strips—the adult can be one character and your child another.	• Have your child help you interpret the story, it's his story, too!	• Search for the YouTube video of *Going on a Bear Hunt* performed by the author, Michael Rosen.
• Use books that are repetitive and/or predictable to encourage child participation during book reading.	• Photocopy book illustrations (reduce size, if needed) and leave room for the child to add his own words to the images.	• Even if a child does not want to get up and role-play, they can sit and create gestures to represent story events and actions.
• Children may also be more apt to copy an adult model when intonation is used (particularly when books have repeated words and phrases).	• Or, transcribe the child's story— handwrite or use Post-It notes to quickly add text to a page.	

Source: Reproduced with permission of the author Anne Spitler-Kashuba (2009).

Phonological Awareness

Phonological awareness is the ability to mentally manipulate words, syllables, and sounds of spoken language. Cabell et al. (2009) defined phonological awareness as "an umbrella term that refers to children's metalinguistic understandings about the sound structure of language . . . [and] appears to develop in a general sequence: rhyme, alliteration, words, syllables, onset-rime, and phoneme" (p. 5). The relationship between phonological awareness and later reading and spelling abilities is well documented (Goldsworthy, 2003, and Gillon, 2004, for example). Torgesen and Mathes (2000) pointed out that "phonological awareness is most commonly defined as one's sensitivity to, or explicit awareness of, the phonological structure of words in one's language. In short, it involves the ability to notice, think about, or manipulate the individual sounds in words" (p. 2). Because of their unique background in phonology, phonetics, and child language disorders, speech and language specialists are perfectly positioned to serve as a critical member of the educational team assessing and treating language-based reading problems. Butler (1999) noted that "SLPs and other language specialists whose training and experience prepare them to support both oral and written language prevention and intervention can play pivotal roles, particularly in school-based settings" (p. iv). Lyon (1997) maintained that speech-language specialists are "gems" in integrating phonological awareness into reading stating "they know how to interpret the data, know the importance of phonological awareness . . . [and] need to explicitly and daily translate what they know about language and reading to teachers" (p. 5).

Suggestions for Working on Phonological Awareness

The role of the speech-language specialist in literacy has long been a research and clinical area of interest to me, and I refer the reader of this resource to several earlier publications. In *Developmental Reading Disabilities: A Language Based Treatment Approach* (2003), I detailed the role of speech-language pathology in the area of oral and written literacy. In that book, I outlined a phonological awareness treatment approach with suggested materials. I have included some of the recommended goals from that text here under the following headings: implicit and explicit teaching at the word, syllable, and sound level (see Chapter 4 of this resource for a discussion of implicit and explicit teaching). The following activities are suggested.

1. **To increase phonological awareness at the word level: implicit teaching**

   Reading Aloud. Choose a wide variety of books including wordless books such as those by Mayer such as *Frog, Where Are You?* (1969), *A Boy, A Dog, A Frog, and a Friend* (1971), and *Frog Goes to Dinner* (1974), or books by Turk such as *Happy Birthday Max* (1984a), and *Max Packs* (1984b). Placing sticky notes on pages as you and the child tell a story about the pictures draws attention to the spoken words that are put into print on a page in a book.

   Reading books with pictures inserted in lines of print such as *P. B. Bear's Birthday Party* (Davis, 1984) provides additional opportunities to draw attention to words that can be "read" by naming the pictures. In this particular book, P. B. Bear (picture of a teddy bear) is introduced. "The P. stands for pajamas, because his (picture of pajamas) are his favorite clothes. (picture of a bed) time is his favorite time of day." You read the words and the child "reads" the pictures.

2. **To increase phonological awareness at the word level: explicit teaching**

   Identifying Words and Sentences. As you read to a child point to various words and say: "This word says 'HELLO,' that's what the boy said to the farmer." Explain there are words in sentences and that sentences end with marks say as this "dot. It ends the sentence." Show the child how words are separated on the page by the spaces between them.

   Filling in Words as Adult Reads. After you read a book a few times to a child, begin to omit words as you read asking that the child fill in the word. Books with repetitive phrases are excellent sources for this such as *Going on a Bear Hunt* (Rosen, 1989) where you repeat, "We can't go over it, we can't go under it, we have to go through it." Reinforce the child directly with "you are filling in the words."

Counting Words Heard. After a child is familiar with a book ask him/her to count the number of words he or she hears/ sees as you read from a book. Provide manipulatives such as wooden/plastic blocks to represent the words so the child can count them and tell you the number of words/blocks counted.

3. To increase phonological awareness at the syllable level: implicit teaching

Reading Aloud. As you read to a child occasionally, point to specific words explaining that words are made up of parts, sometimes one, two, three, and so on, and give examples. Sara Ball's mini flip-flap books are excellent sources for children to discover that books are fun and that words have parts. In *Por-gua-can* (1985b), for instance, the pictured porcupine is in three parts with the word parts printed on the left page: por cu pine. When the child turns the top part of the pictured porcupine the left side shows "I" (short /I/ sound) and on the right side there is the pictured head of an iguana and the picture parts on the right make up the Icupine. When the middle section is turned, the left side says "gua" and the right side pictures the trunk of the iguana and the pictured parts on the right now are Iguapine. After turning the bottom part of the page, the print on the left says "na" and the right side is now the completed iguana. Ball's second source includes this same manipulation of printed word and pictures in her flip-flap book *Crocuphant* (1985a).

In the book *Pets in Trumpets*, Most (1991) cleverly shows how words can be broken into parts with pictures and sentences including the following:

"Why did the musician find a dog in his trumpet?"

"Because he always finds a pet in his trum<u>pet</u>."

"What happens when a greedy gorilla eats too many bananas?"

"Greedy gor<u>ill</u>a gets ill." Draw the child's attention to words "hidden" in words (e.g., "pet" in "trumpet" and "ill" in gorilla).

Many books emphasize syllables in words. In *Jamberry* (Degen, 1983), a boy and a bear have fun in a world of berries. "One berry Two berry Pick me a blueberry. Hatberry, shoeberry, in my canoeberry. Three berry, four berry, hayberry. Strawberry." And Mosel's (1968) *Tikki Tikki Tembo*: "Tikki Tikki Tembo No Sa Rembo Chari Bari Ruchi Pip Peri Pembo" provides "syllable-rich" text.

4. To increase phonological awareness at the syllable level: explicit teaching

Differentiating Real Compound Words from Nonreal, Compound Words. The child is asked to indicate when a word is "real," for example, "Is football a word?" Is "ballfoot a word?"

Identifying the Missing Syllable. Show the child two pictures such as "butter" and "fly" and ask him/her to name which one is missing when you remove one, for example "fly." When the child no longer needs the pictures remove them and repeat this without pictures.

Syllable Counting. Ask the child to count the number of syllables in words as you read words. Use blocks if the child needs tangible manipulatives to help count.

Syllable Adding and Deleting. The child is asked to say a word and then to add or delete part of the word. For instance, the child is asked to say "butter" and to add "fly" to it; or to say "butterfly," then to leave out a specified part of the word, for example, "don't say butter," or "don't say fly."

Defining Syllables. The child is taught that words can be divided into parts called "syllables."

Identifying the Common (Hidden) Syllable in Words. The child is asked to identify if a certain syllable is in a word, for example, "Is the word 'cup' in the word 'cupcake?'" "Is it in teacup?" "Is it in hotdog?"

Substituting a Syllable. Ask the child to substitute (replace) a part of a word, for example: Say "horsefly;" instead of "fly" say "butter."

Reversing Syllables in Compound Words. Ask the child to switch word parts, for example, "Switch the two parts of 'baseball'" (ballbase)

5. To increase phonological awareness at the phoneme level: implicit teaching

Reading Aloud. As in the previous goals for phonological awareness training, use books this time emphasizing sounds in words.

In *Double Trouble in Walla Walla* (Clements, 1997) Lulu tells her teacher "But I'm not trying to flip-flop chit-chat. I just have an itty-bitty problem with my homework." Mrs. Bell scowled. "All right for you, Lulu. If you're going to shilly-shally and dilly-dally with all this fancy-schmancy yak-yak, then we will just have to trit-trot down to the principal's office."

In *Pets in Trumpets* (Most, 1991) some words change by emphasizing all the letters except the first one: "Why did the witch let children hold her broomstick? Because the Witch had a very bad itch."

Books with alliteration contain words with repeated first sounds. A wonderful example comes from *Anamalia* (Base, 1986):

Great green gorillas growing grapes in a gorgeous glass greenhouse.

Ingenious iguanas improvising an intricate impromptu on impossibly impractical instruments.

Other books simply have beautiful descriptions of sounds. An example is *Listen to the Rain*, by Martin and Archambault (1988).

"Listen to the rain the roaring pouring rain, the tiptoe pitter-patter, the splish and splash and splatter, the steady sound, the singing of the rain."

6. To increase phonological awareness at the phoneme level: explicit teaching

Blending sounds in monosyllabic words divided into onset-rime beginning with two consonant cluster. Ask the child to combine sounds to make a word, for example, "Say /st/ /op/."

Blending sounds in monosyllabic words divided into onset-rime beginning with a single consonant. Ask the child to combine sounds to make a word, for example, "c + at."

Producing rhyme using content words. Ask the child to make up a word that rhymes with a word you say, for example, "Tell me a word that rhymes with 'dog.'"

Matching rhyme. Ask the child to identify which of three words rhymes with a word you say (e.g., "Which word rhymes with 'hat'? 'sat,' 'cow,' 'sheep'"?)

Sound matching. Ask the child to guess which of two to four words begin with a particular sound, for example, "Which two words begin with /k/: cow, book, coat, pig?"

Blending three continuous sounds to form a monosyllabic word. Ask the child to put sounds together to make a word, e.g. "say sssss-uuuuh—mmmmm. Choose words beginning with continuant sounds, for example, /m/, /n/, /s/, /f/, /sh/, /th/, /r/, /h/, /l/, and /w/.

Blending three noncontinuous sounds to form a monosyllabic word. Ask the child to put sounds together to make a word (e.g., "say d-ah-g.?"). Choose words beginning with noncontinuant sounds, for example, /p/, /b/, /t/, /d/, k/, and /g/.

Supplying the Initial or Final Sound. Ask the child to tell you what sound is missing in a word, for example, "phone, own. What sound is missing in 'own' that you hear in phone?" (/f/). "What sound is missing in 'how' that you hear in 'house'?"

Judging the Initial or Final Sound Same. Ask the child to tell you which of three to four words begins/ends with the same sound heard in the beginning/end of a stimulus word. For example, "Which word begins with the same first sound you hear in 'car'?: 'boat,' 'rat,' 'cow'" "Which word ends with the same last sound you hear in 'walk'?: 'track,' 'flower,' 'boat'?"

Counting Sounds in Words. Ask the child to count all sounds in a word. Begin with two-sound monosyllabic words. For example, "How many sounds do you hear in the word 'be?'"

Deleting the Initial or Final Sound. Ask the child to leave out the first or last sound of a word, for example, "Say 'stop' without /s/," or "Say 'boat' without /t/."

Substituting Sounds in Words. Ask the child to substitute a sound in a word, e.g., "Say 'skip.' Instead of /k/ say /l/."

Saying Words Backward or Sound Reversing. Ask the child to say words backward, for example, "say 'cat' backward." (tack)

Switching First Sounds in Words. Ask the child to switch the first sounds in two words, for example, "If we switch the first sounds in 'big hat' the new words are 'hig bat.'"

Learning a "Secret Language," for example, "Pig Latin." Ask the child to put the first consonant of a word at the end and add a long /a/ sound, for example, "table" becomes "abletay."

Because of my belief in using contextualized materials in our training (see Chapter 4) I wrote two and co-authored a third *Sourcebook of Phonological Awareness Activities* books (see Goldsworthy, 1998, 2000, and Goldsworthy & Pieretti, 2004). In the first two books, some of the classic children's books were chosen such as *Gingerbread Boy, Goldilocks, Jack and the Beanstalk, Snow White, Blueberries for Sal, Corduroy, Stone Soup, Three Pigs, Hungry Thing, Very Hungry Caterpillar*, and *Harry the Dirty Dog*. The third book included books preferred by older students such as the Harry Potter books, *Tom Sawyer, Charlotte's Web, Little House on the Prairie*, and *Amelia Bedilia*. The phonological awareness activities described in this section at the word, syllable, and sound levels plus many more were included in the three sourcebooks using words from the books selected.

Print Awareness

Print awareness has to do with how children understand "how print works in a book. This knowledge includes: print conventions (e.g., print is read from left to right and top to bottom on a page); print functions (e.g., print carries meaning); and print forms (e.g., letters make up words)" (Cabell et al., 2009). Gillon (2004) suggested that developing toddlers' print awareness "helps build a strong foundation from which phonological awareness can emerge" (p. 59). Specifically, Gillon recommended "drawing (toddlers') attention to words in the environment (stop signs, exit signs, advertising signs) and to the meaning of large, clear print in storybooks. For example, pointing to the words while reading the title of a storybook; finding the main character's name each time it appears in print (assuming the use of large print in a children's book), and bringing the child's attention to the initial letter(s) and sounds in the character's name; observing how rhyming words often look the same and sound the same at the ends of words in rhyme stories such as Dr. Seuss's *The Cat in the Hat* (p. 59). In their discussion of accelerating preschoolers' early literacy development, Cabell et al. (2009) explained that print knowledge is "a multidimensional construct that refers to an array of understandings that emerge for many children before formal reading instruction" (p. 68).

Suggestions for Working on Print Awareness: Implicit Teaching

I like to have materials in my room that will facilitate the child's growing awareness of print. Included among these materials are:

- Paper and crayons, markers, pencils, and water color paints and brushes to draw or paint people or objects or whatever the child wants to draw.
- Paper on which to practice printing the alphabet, names of family members, and so on.
- Sticky notes or paper and tape to write notes to display on walls or refrigerators.
- A small metal post office box with a movable signal to indicate that the box has mail. Write notes with the child's name on them and place in the mailbox or in small envelopes in the mailbox. Have the child read the mail and print an answer to then be placed in the mailbox.
- Just let children explore the materials in the beginning. Don't teach yet. They may want to draw the sun and a house, their family, copy from a box in your room, print their names. Just let this happen without much direction.

Suggested Materials

Wordless Books. *Examples:* A number of Boy/Frog books such as *Frog Goes to Dinner* (Mayer, 1974), and any of the *Max* books (Turk, 1981).

Suggestions on How to Use: Allow the child to explore each material. Encourage her/him to look at the various pictures in the book and comment about the fact that there are no words! Then tell the child that he or she can make up a story about the pictures using his or her words, which you will print on sticky notes and apply to however many pages the student wants to "talk about." In this way, you encourage the child to tell a story about the pictures and that the words going into the book are his or hers. Encourage the child to ask for "the book with his or her words" on his or her next visit. When I have inadvertently taken a child's sticky notes out of the book, I have been admonished by that child on his or her next visit with: "Why don't you have my words/story in this book? They were here last week!" In *Frog Goes to Dinner*, the child can make up a story about the pictures such as the following. A boy goes to dinner with his family. He has a frog in his pocket. The frog jumps into the sax, falls out on the man's head, and jumps into the food. The man chases the frog and makes the family leave. The boy laughs with his frog. Likewise, using the *Max* series, sticky notes or other small notes can be used to write down the student's words. For instance, in *Max the Artlover*, (Turk, 1981), the child can tell you that Max takes a nap, goes to an art place, looks at the pictures, chooses a picture of various cheeses, and brings the picture home to hang on his wall.

Books with Some Words Printed Larger. Books with some words that are printed larger than others allow the adult to call attention to "words." Frequently, children will say "but I don't know how to read yet," to which the adult can respond, "Oh I know that, and that's why I'm going to read the words to you. Your job will be to turn the pages." With this indirect, implicit approach to increasing print awareness, the child is being introduced to notions about print and that words can stand by themselves. Explicit instruction follows later.

In *Splat the Cat* (Scotton, 2008), Splat goes to Cat School. Throughout the book, some words are highlighted in larger, bolded print. For example, when Splat gets to school his teacher says: "Everyone, this is Splat. Let's welcome him into our class," said Mrs. Wimpydimple. On the next page in very large print are the words "**Hi, Splat!**" When it's milk time the cats yell "**Hurray!**" In *Dinosaurumpus* (Mitton, 2002), dinosaurs' names are in large bold print such as **Pteranodon** and **Stegosaurus**, as are the sounds they make, for example, **Eeeeek!** And **Clatter! Clatter! Clatter!**

Books with Something Hidden. *Examples:* The *Where's Waldo* books (Hanford, n.d.), and *Highlights* magazines for students are good for this. Encourage children to use their eyes to find hidden objects. Give them hints such as, "Waldo is on the right side of the book this time" indicating with your hand which side is the right side.

Books with Movable Parts. *Examples: The Jolly Postman, or Other People's Letters* (Ahlbergs 1986). Allow the child to explore the material. Let her or him open the envelope pages in *The Jolly Postman* book and remove the cards within. Children have told me "don't read the book . . . just read the letters." There is something magical and fun in opening the envelopes and talking about what's inside. *The Jolly Pocket Postman* (Ahlberg & Ahlberg, 1995) begins with "Once upon a summer's morning, The Jolly Postman woke up yawning, cooked his breakfast, fed the dog, read the paper, and kissed the frog." Then he is off to deliver the mail but has an accident. Throughout the rest of the book, there are pages that are envelopes with letters to the postman. These engage the child to take the letters out of envelopes asking the adult to read the words. Letters inside the envelopes in the Jolly Postman books are too difficult for young children to read. Adding in sticky notes or small pieces of paper with the child's name on them personalizes the notes in a very special way. For example, in one envelope the child can reach into an envelope with a note to him or her from the Three Bears. An additional material to add in at this time is the small metal mailbox (mentioned previously) in which you and the child can place very small cards or pieces of paper on which you have written letters, words, or drawn pictures to be "mailed back," for instance, to the Three Bears.

Sara Ball's mini flip-flap books are excellent sources for children to discover that books are fun and that words have parts. In *Por-gua-can* (1985), and *Crocuphant* (1985) children discover word parts for different animals (see Phonological Awareness at the syllable level).

Books with Printed Words Hidden Behind Flaps. *Examples:* In books such as *Where's Spot* objects and words are hidden under flaps and children typically love to lift the flaps to see what lies beneath. In *Where's Spot* (Hill, 1980), Sally's search for Spot takes her to a number of locations such as behind the door, inside the clock, in the piano, and under the stairs. On these and similar pages the child lifts up the liftable part of the page such as the door, clock, piano and staircase to find animals other that Spot. The "hidden" animals have "talk bubbles" next to them with the word "no" inside the bubble.

Similarly, in *I Know An Old Lady Who Swallowed a Fly* (Hawkins & Hawkins, 1987), the lady's tummy becomes progressively fuller as she swallows item by item. The book begins with "I know an old lady who swallowed a spider that wriggled and jiggled and tickled inside her." When you lift up the lady's apron, you see a fly saying, "My! Oh! My! What a nice place for a fly." As she swallows items, she becomes fuller and fuller until, alas, she sneezes.

In *Peekaboo, Stretch* (Pandell, 2006), two girls want to play peekaboo with their dog, Stretch, who gets into trouble digging holes in the family's yard. The clever drawings delight students, for instance, when one girl says "Peekaboo, Stretch! I see your tail" pictured under the gate. When the child lifts the gate, she or he discovers that what was pictured as Peekaboo's tail is part of a garden hose. Similarly, on another page, one of the girls says "Peekaboo, Stretch! I see your nose," which turns out to be part of a garden glove when the door to cabinet is opened.

Are You There Bunny, I'll Find You, Kitty, and *Out You Come, Mouse* (Powell & Jones, 2002a, 2002b, 2002c) are particularly good for little hands and readers because each book is constructed of thick cardboard and is four pages in length. Each page has a movable part with words behind it. For example, in *Bunny*, the mouse asks "Are you there Bunny?" The child is encouraged to move a part of the page, in this case the rock in front of a cave, to discover a mother bear and her cub with the printed words, "No, Bears live in caves, not bunnies." Students enjoy moving these parts and because the books are so short, in no time, students are "reading" the printed page and the words behind the movable parts. *I'll Find You, Kitty* (Powell & Jones, 2002b) has large bold words on each of five pages. For instance: "Is that **Kitty** behind the scarecrow?" By moving a part under the scarecrow, the single word answer, "No!" is revealed. Likewise "Is that **Kitty** in the trashcan?" is followed by the answer, "NO!" hidden by a movable part. You can ask the child to count the words on the page as well as the word(s) under the movable part(s). Reinforce the child with something like, "Great job, you are counting words!" Don't dare move the movable part by yourself! You'll hear about it!

Books with Words in Print to Be Manipulated. *Example: Word Magic: Magnetic Sentence Builder* (Burrows, n.d.) is a unique way of encouraging a child to experience words as separate and movable. Seven short one-page stories are presented with a sentence about each with three missing words per page. There is a small box containing printed word blocks and you can preselect the words that go with each page. For example, the story about the cat reads The (blank) wears a (blank) on the (blank). You can read the "word blocks" to the child and initially place the blocks above the book. In this story, the word blocks include "cat," "hat," and "mat," which are also printed on the page with a colorful cat wearing a hat on a mat. The child selects which word block goes into the word blanks. Soon they are "reading" each page. When the child knows the words for each page, a word game can be played by inserting incorrect word blocks into the blanks. For example, the cat story can incorrectly read: "The mat wears a cat on the hat." You can model this and then the child can come up with his or her own version demonstrating the ability to move words around and put them in the correct or incorrect places.

Books with Pictured Items Embedded Within Print. *Examples:* In *P. B. Bear's Birthday Party* (Davis, 1994), pictured items are frequently inserted in printed sentences. "Meet P.B. Bear (pictured bear). The P. stands for Pajama, because his (pictured pajamas) are his favorite clothes. (pictured bed) time is his favorite time of day. One morning, (pictured bear) woke up early . . . " The student is asked to "read" the pictured items as you read the text. Reinforce the student for helping you read the book.

Rebus Read-Along Stories such as *Inside a Barn in the Country* (Capucilli 1995) cleverly inserts increasing numbers of pictured items throughout the book. The book begins with "Here is a barn in the country. Here is the mouse that squeaked in the hay inside a barn in the country." On the next page the sentence reads, "Here is the (picture of mouse) that squeaked in the hay and woke up the horse that whinnied neigh inside a barn in the country." Several pages later: "Here is the (pictured mouse) that squeaked in the hay and woke up the (pictured horse) that whinnied neigh that woke up the (pictured cow) that started to moo that woke up the (pictured rooster) cock-a-doodle-doo that woke up the (pictured chicks) that started to peep that woke up a couple of sleepy white (pictured sheep)." You read the words and the child names the pictures as well as fills in the repetitive phrases such as "inside a barn in the country."

Another of Capucilli's (1998) clever books, *Inside a House That Is Haunted*, begins with "Here is a house that is haunted. . . . Here is the (pictured hand) that knocked on the door and startled the spider that dropped to the floor inside a house that is haunted." Several pages later the book reads: "Here is the (pictured hand) that knocked on the door and startled the (pictured spider) that dropped to the floor that frightened the (pictured ghost) who awoke and cried, 'Boo!' surprising the (pictured cat) that jumped and screeched, 'MEW!' that shook up the (pictured bats) that swooped through the air and jolted the (pictured owl) that called 'Who-Who's there?' that spooked the (pictured mummy) who ran with a shriek rattling the skeleton who moved with a creak inside a house that is haunted." The child benefits from the redundancy of the story line, names the pictured items on each page, and will soon be saying the repeated phrase "inside a house that is haunted." Reinforce the child with "thanks for helping me read this book."

Carle's *The Secret Birthday Message* (1998) cleverly uses pictured geometric and other shapes to tell a story about a boy named Tim who receives a strange envelope under his pillow on his birthday. On the first page, a half circle is shown above the sentence "When the moon comes up" and a pictured star appears on the second page above the printed sentence, "Look for the biggest star." Each page follows with a pictured item including the last page with a pictured rectangle above the printed sentences: "You will see an opening. Climb up and through. That's where you'll find your birthday gift!" A cutout rectangle appears on the next page where the eyes of a puppy appear.

Books with Patterning and Repetition. *Examples: We're Going on a Bear Hunt* (Rosen, 1989) contains delightful words that children enjoy repeating. An example of the patterned, repetitive script: "We're going on a bear hunt. We're going to catch a big one. What a beautiful day. We're not scared." After you have read this book to the child two or three times, ask him or her to fill in more and more of the words. For example, read, "We're going on a bear hunt. We're going to catch a big one. What a beautiful _____" And the next

time you read: "We're going on a bear hunt. We're going to catch a
_____," each time encouraging the child to fill in words you omit.
Children seem to pay particular attention to pages with words
depicting noises heard as a family makes its way through grass,
mud, a river, a snowstorm, a forest, and a cave. For example, the
words used when the family goes through the mud—SQUELCH,
SQUERCH, SQUELCH, SQUERCH—provide an opportunity for the
child to point to each word as it is read. Or as the family goes
through the grass—SWISHY SWASHY SWISHY SWASHY! As before,
after reading these the first few times to the child, begin reading
only part of the words and omitting the last one or two. In no time,
the child is saying these words as you read the book to him or her.

A similar repetition of magic words is found in Martin and
Archambault's (1988) *Listen to the Rain*. There is a melody to the
words in this book with a combination of repetition, alliteration, and
rhyme. The following example illustrates: "Listen to the rain, the
singing of the rain, the tiptoe pitter-patter, the splish and splash and
splatter leaving all outdoors a muddle, a mishy mushy muddy puddle."

The repetition of the word "berry" stands out in Degen's (1983)
Jamberry. For example, "One berry Two berry Pick me a blueberry.
Hatberry Shoeberry In my canoeberry." Children delight in the
illustrations with corresponding printed words "Raspberry rabbits,
Brasberry band, Elephants skating on raspberry jam."

In *The Napping House* (Wood, 1984), the child discovers the
repetition of "in a napping house, where everyone is sleeping"
throughout the book. The book begins with, "There is a house, a
napping house, where everyone is sleeping. And in that house
there is a bed, a cozy bed in a napping house, where everyone is
sleeping." Simple enough! But alas! Before long, the snoring granny
is layered with a dreaming child, a dozing dog, a snoozing cat, a
slumbering mouse, and a wakeful flea always in a napping house
where everyone is sleeping until the end. Once again, repeated
readings typically result in the child filling in words and phrases as
you "read the book together."

Suggestions for Working on Print Awareness:
Explicit Teaching

Marvin and Wright (1997) found that parents of children with language impairment were less likely to ask questions when reading
aloud to their children, comment on nonprint activities, or interact

in oral story telling with their children. Furthermore, children with language impairment were less likely than children with other disabilities to "listen to stories or ask or answer questions of an adult who is reading aloud. These findings suggest that literacy socialization (i.e., interaction with and exposure to early experiences with print) and language impairment have a symbiotic relationship such that the presence of language impairment may negatively affect children's meaningful engagement with print" (Lovelace & Stewart, 2007). Justice and Ezell (2001) found that, the more a child interacts with print in meaningful ways, the more he or she knows how print works in books.

Lovelace and Stewart (2007) summarized an approach identified by Justice and Kaderavek (2004) that integrates aspects of explicit teaching (see Chapter 4) "used to direct a child's attention to literacy targets through the use of direct, sequenced instructional opportunities with aspects of an embedded approach where adults serve as facilitators of children's literacy learning" (p. 6). The researchers described two methods that have emerged as useful strategies during shared book reading, "which suggests that an embedded-explicit model of intervention may be effective in helping children acquire early literacy knowledge concurrently with oral language" (p. 6). *Dialogic reading* involves an "adult asking questions, providing feedback, and structuring responses that allow children to participate at their skill level" during a reading aloud activity (p. 6). *Explicit print referencing* intervention is structured to enhance children's print awareness. In this intervention, the adult directs children's attention to print concepts embedded in book reading through verbal and nonverbal cues (Justice & Ezell, 2004). *Prompts* or *evocative techniques* used during explicit print referencing involve the adult asking questions and making requests about prompts that require the child to respond. *Nonevocative strategies* involve "nonverbal references (that) include pointing to print and tracking print" and do not require a child to respond (p. 7). In their study of increasing print awareness in preschoolers with language impairment, Lovelass and Stewart (2007) found that children with language impairment require implementation of a systematic, explicit print referencing procedure and that "when the children engaged in twice weekly, shared book reading . . . without explicit print referencing . . . knowledge of print concepts did not improve" (p. 22). Some of the explicit print referencing techniques used are summarized in Table 5–3.

Table 5–3. Techniques for Increasing Print Awareness in Preschoolers with Language Impairment Using Nonevocative Print Referencing by Lovelace and Stewart (2007)

BOOK CONVENTIONS		
Concepts	*What Adult Does*	*Acceptable Child Response*
1. **Illustration**	Show child page with illustration. Say "Show me an illustration."	Points to picture
2. **Print**	Show child page with illustration and print. Say "Show me the print."	Points to print
3. **Page**	Turn to page in book. Say "Show me a page in the book."	Grasps/points to page
4. **Front/back of book**	Show child front/back of book. Say "Give book upside down and backward." Say "Show me front of the book." Say "Show me back of the book."	Rights book and shows front of it Points/shows back of book
5. **Author/ Illustrator**	Show title page. Say "This is the author's/illustrator's name. What does 'author/illustrator' mean?"	S/he wrote/drew pictures for the book
6. **Top/bottom of book**	Say "Show me top/bottom of book."	Points to top/bottom of book
7. **Book Title**	Say "Show me the title of the book."	Points to title on book/cover

PRINT CONVENTIONS		
Concepts	*What Adult Does*	*Acceptable Child Response*
1. **Begin reading**	Show page with print and say "Show me where I begin reading."	Points to 1st line
2. **1st line print next page**	Find print on both left/right pages. Ask "Where do I go next to keep reading?"	Points to 1st line next page
3. **Left/right of page**	Show child page asking "Which way should I go to read this page?"	Gestures left to right on page

Table 5–3. *continued*

PRINT CONVENTIONS

Concepts	What Adult Does	Acceptable Child Response
4. **Top/bottom of page**	Show child page asking "Where do I go next to keep reading?"	Gestures top to bottom on page
5. **Beginning/end of story**	Give book to child. Say "Show me beginning/end of the story."	Opens book and points to 1st/last pages

PRINT FORM/PRINT CONVENTION

Concepts	What Adult Does	Acceptable Child Response
1. **1st/last letters**	Show child page with print. Say "Show me 1st/last letter of a word."	Points to 1st/last letters of any word.

PRINT FORM

Concepts	What Adult Does	Acceptable Child Response
1. **Letter/word**	Show child page with print. Say "Show me one letter/word."	Points to just one letter/word

Alphabet Knowledge

Cabell et al. (2009) explained that "alphabet knowledge includes children's understandings of the shapes, names, and sounds of the letters of the alphabet. This includes knowledge of upper- and lowercase letters" (p. 5). These authors cited other researchers noting that among preschoolers and kindergartners "the ability to identify letter names is one of the strongest unique predictors of later reading achievement" (p. 5).

Suggestions for Working on Alphabet Knowledge

The Chicka Chicka ABC Magnet Book (Martin & Archambault, 2002) offers an outstanding source of discovery through repetition, rhyme, and intrigue with plastic letters. Read the story to a child and allow him or her to place the plastic letters that accompany the book on the corresponding page. The letters will adhere to the magnetic sheet that can be moved to rest behind each of the book pages. For example, the first page reads "A told B, and B told C, 'I'll meet you at the top of the coconut tree.'" A coconut tree is pictured with the lowercase letters: a, b, and c. After you read the words, the child can place the magnetic plastic letters on top of the printed letters on the page. After each page, the child can remove the letters and put them into a can or box. At the end of the book, there is a page for the child to create his or her own words or scenes with the magnetic letters. All the letters of the alphabet are printed on the last page and the child can place the magnetic letters on each of these.

In *Alphabet Soup* (Banks, 1988), a little boy did not want his lunch and shouts, "I won't eat it!" His mother says, "My, you're as grumpy as a bear," and the boy dips his spoon into his soup and growls, spelling B-E-A-R." The book continues with the boy imagining a wonderful adventure with a bear. They meet an ogre who won't let them pass by so the boy dips into his soup and spells S-W-O-R-D and the ogre lets them pass by. The boy and the bear come to a lake and the bear says "I can't swim," and the boy dips his spoon into his soup and spells "B-O-A-T" and they float away The adventure continues with the boy spelling more words in his alphabet soup such as "net," " rope," " tree," "cage," " house," and "bed."

In the *Alphabet Mystery* (Wood & Wood, 2003), Little " x" has disappeared from Charley's Alphabet. All the other letters go on an adventure to try and locate "x." The story begins with "Every night, the little letters from Charley's Alphabet tuck themselves into bed. And every night, just for fun, each one calls out his name. 'a-b-c-d-e-f-g-h-i-j-k-l-m-n-o-p-q-r-s-t-u-v-**w**-_-y-z!' But tonight, something is wrong. Who didn't say his name?" The rest of the letters hop onto a pencil and set off zooming over cities, towns, and fields in search of "x." In the middle of the story, the letters think they have found Little "x." "When they landed at a castle, a heavy door creaked open. In a voice as creaky as the door, a crooked Capital [I] said, 'Who dares to visit the Master's castle in the middle of the night?' Brave Little [b] spoke up: 'We've come to solve a mystery. Have you seen Little x?' 'Follow me,' Crooked [I] said, 'but don't wake the Master, or you'll be alphabet soup!'" The book ends with [x] returning home with his friends and learning the importance of being an "x" as on mom's birthday cake to indicate "kisses."

Think-It-Through Materials (1979) is an intriguing material to present to children who are aware of printed letters and who are interested in beginning reading and writing. In *Think-It-Through Beginning Reading Visual Discrimination* Book 1, children are introduced to the concept of matching objects on the left page with objects on the right page. For instance, letter approximations (e.g., l) are matched with the same presentation on the right. Also included in this first book are matchups for lines presented in different directions, determining which pictured item would come next in a pattern, determining objects turned in the same direction, matching small letters, matching capital letters, matching sequence patterns of objects and then letters, and finally matching two-letter pairs, for example, "on" "um" "gn" and "rn" with corresponding two-letter pairs on the right side of the book. In all of the *Think-It-Through* books, the child places a plastic tile in a case each time he or she chooses a visual letter or picture. At the conclusion of each exercise, the child closes the case, turns it upside down, and opens it to see if the colored design matches the design on the page she or he has just completed. Children frequently come into the Center asking "Can we please do the blue thing with the letters so I can get the matchup?" As with all the *Think-It-Through* materials, children learn as they are having fun.

Games such as UpWords (1997) is a word game designed for 8-year-olds to adults. However, it can be used with younger children as a reinforcer by "spelling" little words matching those they may be encountering in their early reading. For instance, if the child has read the word "cat" this word can be spelled with tiles on the game board that comes with UpWords. By preselecting other beginning letters of the "-at" family or phonogram, the clinician provides an opportunity for the child to spell other –at words by stacking other letters, for example. r, s, p, f, and so on on top of the "c" letter on the board.

Using letter cubes found in games such as *Boggle Jr.* (1992) adds to the fun of learning alphabet letter names and how to spell simple words. *Boggle Jr.* contains 8 plastic letter squares and 30 color picture/word cards. You can make up your own "rules" encouraging your child to choose the letter cubes that match the letters printed on each card under the pictured item. You can carry over this activity to have the child print the letters or words on paper or a whiteboard after spelling out the words with the letter cubes on the plastic tray.

Computer programs such as Curious George (2002) and Ultimate Phonics (2000) are appropriate to add in when a child has shown interest in the alphabet and can be taught how to use the computer mouse and arrow keys. In Curious George, the monkey (George) needs to reconstruct an important note that has accidentally been torn into pieces. The child helps George with this task by playing various games on three levels of difficulty. Level 1 includes activities with uppercase letters, consonants, long vowels, beginning sounds, and simple spelling. An example of one of the games the student is to "play" at this level has Curious George helping to wash windows. The child is asked to, "Listen to the letter George needs." The window washer displays a letter and George must find the matching letter. Level 2 includes upper- and lowercase letters, consonants, short vowels, ending sounds, and spelling. One of the Level 2 activities has George washing windows but this time matches lower- to uppercase letters. Level 3 includes alphabetical order, consonants, long and short vowels, beginning and ending sounds, and spelling. A sample of Level 3 activities includes having the child click on one of five letters a pictured item begins with, and then clicking on each of the letters that follow in the word, each displayed in array of five letters.

When the child moves into beginning reading (see Early Reading and Writing), Ultimate Phonics can be a teaching and reinforcing activity to introduce at this time. The beginning lessons include short A vowel in consonant-vowel-consonant words such as at, am an, ran, rap, can, and Hal. The child can read the word on the computer screen and then click on the printed word to hear the man's voice read it aloud.

Emergent Writing

"Children's earliest writing attempts may include drawing and scribbling. As their knowledge about print grows, they write using letterlike forms. Then they begin to include letters in their writing, usually from their name" (Cabell et al., 2009, p. 6).

Suggestions for Working on Emergent Writing

Stage 1: Random Scribbling (15 months to 2½ Years)

Parrot (2008) noted that at this early age "children are delighted to figure out how to hold a crayon" and recommends the extra jumbo crayons. "Babies and toddlers will usually hold the crayons in a tight fist and use large motions from their shoulders to produce scribbles" (Parrot, 2008, p. 1). Neuman (2004) described early experiments with writing between 18 months to 2 years, suggesting that "children love to explore the movements of pencils, crayons, and markers on paper. But as they get greater control and greater coordination, you start to see that recognizable shapes, lines, and patterns are revealed" (p. 1). When given a crayon or pencil around 1½ years of age the child makes random marks on the paper. Bailer (2003) noted that "marks are often light colored in nature and are the result of banging the drawing tool on paper, dragging, or sweeping . . . (while) the child's attention may be elsewhere as he or she is drawing" (p.1). Bailer pointed out that this "exploratory scribbling" represents the beginning of the child's literacy development" (p. 1) and encourages the adult to make marks on another piece of paper at the child's level, cautioning us to scribble and not to draw a picture. "Provide one drawing utensil at a time to help the child focus his or her attention on the process of scribbling instead of the profusion of colors" (p. 1). Lowenfeld (1987) described scribbling at 2 years of age as "enjoyable kinesthetic activity, not attempts at portraying the visual world . . . Soon they begin to name scribbles, an important milestone in development." In her description of "disordered scribbling, Bailer (2003) suggested that the adult now provides the child with "plenty of experience" in making marks with crayons and paper as well as with finger paint" (p. 2). Young children begin using writing in pretend play. Neuman (2004) explained that "they write orders and checks and make to-do lists all to embellish their dramatic play. These early activities indicate that children are beginning to understand the functions and purposes of print" (p. 1).

Stage 2: Controlled Scribbling (2–3 Years)

During this time children frequently transition to holding a crayon between their thumb and pointer finger. "Their scribbles may show more repeated marks or patterns such as spirals, open circles, curved lines, and straight lines. As their muscle control develops, toddlers will enjoy experimenting with using a paintbrush, or working with model clay" (Parrot, 2008, p. 1).

Stage 3: Lines and Patterns (2½–3½ Years)

Lowenfeld (1987) described the "preschematic stage" at age 3 years as the first conscious creation of form and noted that this allows us a window into the child's thinking process." Edwards (1999) described this stage of symbols as making the discovery of art . . . ," a drawn symbol can stand for "something out there in the environment. The child makes a circular mark, looks at it, adds two marks for eyes, points to the drawing, and says, 'Mommy,' or 'Daddy,' or 'That's me,' or 'My dog'" (p. 71). Edwards noted that by 3½ imagery in art becomes more complex reflecting children's growing world awareness and perceptions. "A body is attached to the head, though it may be smaller than the head. Arms may still grow out of the head, but more often they emerge from the body—sometimes from below the waist. Legs are attached to the body" (pp 71-72). Parrot (2008) explained that, "at this stage, children begin to understand that writing consists of special lines and curves that repeat in certain patterns. Very often, children will pretend to write. Although their scribbling may not have any actual letters you may see some early components that make up the alphabet such as "S" like curves, small circles, and sharp lines" (p. 2).

Stage 4: Pictures of Objects and People, Pictures That Tell Stories (3–5 Years)

During this stage, children often produce unplanned artwork and, after they are finished, they will decide what it is, for example, "It's Grandma." As Parrot (2008) explained, "eventually, you may notice your child thinking about what she will draw before committing crayon to paper. This is an important developmental milestone. She is now engaged in symbolic thinking! She understands that her artwork can symbolize objects, people, or events" (p. 2). Edwards (1999) noted that by 4 years of age "children are keenly aware of details of clothing—buttons and zippers, for example, appear as details of the drawings. Fingers appear at the ends of arms and hands, and toes at the ends of legs and feet" (p. 72). And 4- and 5-year-olds begin to tell stories in their drawings by adding details such as a child carrying an umbrella or a sister with big teeth in her mouth drawn by her younger brother" (Edwards, 1999, p. 73).

Beaty (2008) emphasized the importance of early scribbling as, "scribbling is to writing what babbling is to speaking: an early stage of children's development that should be encouraged" (p.1). Children tend to scribble in the middle of their paper and then add another line of scribbles beneath the first one and then picture scribbles (described above) become differentiated from writing scribbles. Children frequently pretend to read what they have written or ask the adult to read their "writing" for them. Beaty explained that, when writing, children first see the whole pattern, or the lines across a page, and later they identify separate words and then separate letters. During this "emergent stage," children observe and "seem to extract the broad general features of the writing system—that it is arranged in rows across a page; that it consists of loops, sticks, and connected lines, repeated over and over. Some children fill pages of scribbled lines over and over from top to bottom in a sort of self-imposed practice" (p. 2).

Stage 5: Letter and Word Practice (3–5 Years)

Children now begin writing "real" letters frequently those in their name. "Children also begin to understand that letters fit together in special ways to make words. While they may not be able to write words on their own, they do understand that some words are short and some are long" (Parrot, 2008, p. 2).

To encourage young children to draw and write, Colorado (2008) suggested adults have the following materials available: pencils, crayons, or markers; yarn or ribbon; writing paper or notebook; cardboard or heavy paper; construction paper; and safety scissors. Furthermore, the following ideas were included before getting started:

Provide a place: a desk, table or other area with a smooth, flat surface with good lighting.

Provide the materials: as listed above

Brainstorm: talk with the child about his or her ideas and impressions and encourage him or her to describe people and events to you.

Encourage the child to draw and discuss his or her drawings: as the child draws ask questions such as "What is the boy doing?" "Can you tell a story about this picture?" Write the child's story down as she or he tells it.

Encourage the child to write his or her name: pointing out the letters in his or her name in other places such as on signs, in stores, and so forth.

Turn the child's writing into books: pasting drawings and writings on pieces of construction paper, turning it into a book with title and the child's name as author. Bind the book with yarn or ribbon.

Included among suggestions provided in Reading Is Fundamental (2009) are the following:

Writing tables. All children write best when they have a comfortable place to work. Young children can sit on a child-size chair at a play table cleared of toys. Older children can work at the desk or table where you do your own writing, or desks of their own.

Writing paper. The smallest writers need the largest paper for their drawings and scribbles. Introduce lined paper only when a beginning writer has mastered the alphabet and forms letters that are the same size.

Writing tools. Thick watercolor markers and crayons are best for toddlers' drawings and scribbles. Preschoolers like thin markers, regular crayons, and chalk. Beginning writers need pencils with erasers.

Keyboards. A personal computer can enhance the child's writing experiences. Perfect letters appear at the press of a key—no small miracle for a young child struggling to control a pencil.

Playful activities to encourage preschoolers natural fascination with writing including:
1. *Shopping.* Before going, ask a child to write out a list of things he or she needs.
2. *Props for pretend play.* Given a marker and a pad of paper, little doctors can scribble their prescriptions and

waiters can take orders. Opportunities for playtime writing are endless: restaurant menus, store signs and price tags, tickets for a show or a train ride, and so on. Some children may ask for help in writing real words; others are satisfied with their own marks or drawings.

3. *Post office.* Equip a play post office with paper, envelopes, and cards. Save stickers and stamps from junk mail for pretend postage stamps.

4. *Taking dictation.* Be your child's secretary and take down words he or she tells. You can read these stories back to the child.

5. *Homemade books.* First books are often stories told in pictures on folded pages, perhaps with a few words or captions. You might introduce beginning writers to comic strip format so they can add words in voice bubbles/balloons and thought clouds to their picture stories. Young children also like to make their own A-B-C books by drawing or pasting pictures on pages labeled for each letter of the alphabet.

Early Reading and Writing

Cabell et al. (2009) explained that "once children are systematically using letter sounds to decode words and invent spellings, they are beginning readers in the stage of early literacy development who need very different instruction, particularly in the code-related realm" (p. 4). Children now are moving from "reading" logographs (visual representations of words such as the red hexagon for STOP) and moving into discovering the alphabetic principle, that is, what sounds the letters make. Between the ages of 4 and 7 years, children begin to translate words they hear into letters on paper.

Suggestions for Working on Early Reading and Writing

Some years ago, I read about the work being done at the Center for Reading and Language Research at Tufts University by Wolf, Miller, and Donnelly (2000) known as Retrieval, Automaticity, Vocabulary

Engagement and Orthography (RAVE-O). This program being researched and implemented by classroom teachers struck a chord with me because it so closely resembled the work I was doing as a speech-language pathologist. Three of the primary goals as described by the RAVE-O researchers were:

- RAVE-O's primary goal is the "development of fluency in reading outcome behaviors including word identification, word attack, and comprehension."
- RAVE-O emphasizes the "interconnectedness of lexical and sublexical processes" to facilitate reading."
- RAVE-O's third goal focuses on metalinguistic strategies. Because RAVE-O "is grounded in the belief that word recognition is facilitated by semantic knowledge," core words are selected to use in the sublexical onset-rime activities and again as words to study in multiple meaning activities (p. 377).

Because aspects of this program mirror my own therapy, I began having my master's level speech-language pathology students make modified RAVE-O kits to be used during their child language practicum. The phases of Modified RAVE-O are described below. The "kits" are the components included in the program. A book is selected to read to a child. The kit contains file folders for the following items:

File 1: Phonological awareness materials corresponding with the book you have read to the child are copied and put into this file.

File 2: Core words are selected from the book and pictures of these are placed into this file. The child will be introduced to 5 to 10 core words from the book (fewer if you have selected a shorter book). You should select words that lend themselves to having multiple meanings and that have fairly common word families in them (e.g., -at, -am, -id, -et, -op, etc.). In this file, the child will see the core words and their definitions and is asked to copy the words and/or definitions in the corresponding journal that accompanies the kit. (see File 6)

File 3: Word family cards are kept in this file. On one side of the cards the word is divided into onset and rime with a dash, for example, c-at, and on the other side of the card the word is printed without the dash: cat. For every word family you select, try to make 5 to 8 word family cards (e.g., cat, rat, sat, fat, mat). The child is asked to read the separated rime cards and then the nonseparated words. You can then engage the child in a "sort" activity in which she or he reads each card and places it in separated or nonseparated stacks. The words also should be written in the journal on different "Word Family" pages.

File 4: Core words: multiple meanings. This file contains pictures and short printed definitions of the multiple meanings the core words may have. For instance, "trunk" might be the "trunk of a tree," "a trunk to pack," and an "elephant's trunk." Download pictures from clip art, Google Images, or other picture sites and glue onto sticky notes to place next to the various definitions. In this file you will have "worksheets" with the various multiple word meanings and the child places the Sticky Note with picture next to the correct definition of each core word. These core words with their various definitions can now be copied by the child onto the "Core Words" page in the journal.

File 5: Word webs or other diagrams with each core word in the center and lines drawn out to the printed words "who," "what," "where," "when," and "why." Using the above example, the child is now asked questions about the word "trunk" to extend each of the multiple meanings, for example, "Who would want a trunk?" "What would you put into a trunk?" "Where would you find a trunk?" "When would you use a trunk?" and "Why would you want a trunk?"

File 6: Journal. You can staple several sheets of paper together or buy colorful thin journals to keep in this file for use with various children throughout your work with any particular book.

In an attempt to design a therapy program consistent with ASHA guidelines, Pieretti's (2001) master's thesis at California State University, Sacramento used a modified RAVE-O program to fit the scope and caseload demands of speech-language specialists. It also set out to measure Modified RAVE-O's impact on students as compared with more traditional top-down language therapy such as targeting isolated vocabulary expansion, synonyms and antonyms, listening comprehension, oral vocabulary, and verbal analogies. Six participants, aged 8 years, 7 months to 10 years, 11 months, with identified oral language and reading problems with deficits in both phonological awareness skills and rapid naming abilities, were selected to participate in eight individual 45-minute therapy sessions. Three participants were randomly assigned to the "Modified RAVE-O Therapy Group" and three to the "Traditional Language Therapy Group." Pre- and post-testing scores on the Woodcock Language Proficiency Battery-Revised (WLPB-R) (Woodcock, 1991) and The Comprehensive Test of Phonological Processing (CTOPP) (Wagner, Torgesen, & Rashotte, 1999) provided a level of measurement. Results of this study revealed some important trends:

- The Modified RAVE-O participants increased by more than two times the composite standard score point increases of the Traditional Language Therapy Group on the Phonological Awareness Composite, the Alternate Phonological Awareness Composite and the Phonological Memory Composite of the CTOPP.
- The Modified RAVE-O group demonstrated a seven-point Rapid Naming Composite standard score increase while the Traditional Language Therapy Group showed no improvement in the ability to rapidly name items on the CTOPP.
- The Modified RAVE-O participants demonstrated a marked improvement in the ability to decode words on the Word Attack subtest of the WLPB-R, whereas the Traditional Language group demonstrated a decrease in this ability.
- The Modified RAVE-O group demonstrated more than three times the standard score point increase of the Traditional Language Therapy (TL) group on the Passage Comprehension subtest of the WLPB-R.

The Modified RAVE-O group demonstrated significantly higher standard score point increases on four of five WLPB-R oral language subtests (Table 5–4).

Modified RAVE-O begins by selecting a child's book and reading it to the child two to three times. The child should be able to retell most of the story so that you know she or he is familiar with

Table 5–4. Scores on Five Subtests of WPLB-R Oral Language Subtests for Two Therapy Groups in Pieretti 2001 Study

Subtest of WPLB-R	m-RAVE-O	TL
Listening Comprehension	+14.00	+8.33
Verbal Analogies	+12.67	+4.33
Oral Vocabulary	+11.34	+6.33
Picture Vocabulary	+7.00	+11.67
Memory for Sentences	+5.00	+1.66

words from the story. You want to know this because the first part of Modified RAVE-O is to work on explicit phonological awareness training. Work directed toward phonological awareness is essentially working on the "form" of our language, that is, we are asking a child to listen to and manipulate words, syllables and sounds of words he or she has just heard in the book read to him or her. Pieretti used the activities from *Sourcebook of Phonological Awareness Activities: Children's Classic Literature* (Goldsworthy, 2000). Subsequent activities were based on the RAVE-O curriculum, namely: multiple meaning words, onset-rime word families, word-webbing, and writing in journals. The activities were tied directly to the phonological awareness activities already completed. For example, the multiple meanings of weekly core words were discussed. These words were included in the words used for phonological awareness activities at the word, syllable, and sound levels. Another weekly activity involved choosing three or four rime patterns from these weekly core words (e.g., -ook from book). These, along with two to five new graphemes per week, were printed on onset-rime cards and shown to the participants to pair phonological skills already mastered with orthography.

During each session, the participant printed the ever-increasing number of words on the appropriate rime family/word part page of his/her journal. These words, then, became the basis for the next activity which involved sorting cards imprinted with first hyphenated (b-ook, w-ell, p-op) and then nonhyphenated (book, well, pop) words into rime family/word part stacks. This activity increased in difficulty as weeks progressed as the number of words in the journals increased. Because automaticity is central to RAVE-O, a timed element was added to increase automaticity of reading the rime patterns, namely, participants were instructed to "beat" their previous sorting time. This activity helped prepare participants for later higher level activities involving worksheets on multisyllabic words with the same rime patterns embedded in them. Finally, one word from the core words was chosen each week to use in a word-webbing activity in which in wh-questions were asked about the words selected. The phases of Modified RAVE-O are summarized below.

Phase I: Phonological Awareness Introduced

- *Explicit Phonological Awareness Training:* first 3 to 5 weeks of therapy: using contextualized material from Goldsworthy (1998, 2000) and Goldsworthy and Pieretti (2004) sourcebooks (e.g. *Corduroy, The Little Red Hen*, and *The Three Little Pigs*) These stories are suggested as they coincide with California Elementary curriculum for Language Arts and the Open Court Curriculum.

Phase II: Vocablary Development amd Phonics Fluency

- Review highest level phonological awareness activities
- *Introduce core words for selected stories* (e.g., Jack/Beanstalk: chop, harp
- Begin *orthographic representation of core words:* ask students to give sounds letters make
- Reading and sorting onset-rime cards separated with dashes (word families)

  ch-op   h-arp

  sh-op   sh-arp

  h-op   c-arp

- Reading and sorting onset-rime cards without dashes (word families)

  chop   harp

  shop   sharp

  hop   carp

- *Journals:* students write one word family per journal page
- Generalize onset-rimes: find –op and –arp in bigger words: chopper/ harpsichord
- Multiple meanings of weekly core words: harp = for music; to complain
- Journal: write multiple meanings words and definitions
- Review previous week's definitions
- Multiple meaning word sort

Phase III: Word Webs

- Continue with all steps described in Phase II
- *Word webs on walls:* Ask wh-questions for one or more meanings of each core word
- Journal: copy word webs
- Review previous week's definitions

Phase IV: Review

- Continue with all steps described in Phases II and III
- Review previous week's core word definitions

Phase V: Decoding Print and Fluency

This phase was not part of Pieretti's study but is included in my ongoing therapy with children.

Introduce Simple Decodable Text

In a summary of 30 years of research by the National Institute of Child Health and Human Development (NICHD), Grossen (1997) noted that it is important "to move sequentially from left to right through spellings as children 'sound out,' or say the sound for each spelling" of printed words (p.10). It is helpful for you to model how to sound out words pointing to letters from left to right as you read. This is when I introduce the J & J readers (Greene & Woods, 2000) because they offer a rich source of simple decodable text that slowly progresses into more difficult levels. Children are successful with this series primarily because the books concentrate on short then long vowel sounds affording the novice reader time to be successful with one vowel sound before moving too quickly to the next and the next. It is natural for children to want to look at the pictures in each of the "chapters" in a unit so I suggest that they "take a picture walk with your eyes" before we read.

At the outset I offer a lot of assistance to the child with sounding out and reading words. When we repeat this chapter next session, the child reads more of the words as he or she becomes more proficient with breaking the alphabetic code. The J&J series comes with many resources to build vocabulary, writing and spelling as children progress through the series. Citing others, Cooper (2001) explained that "decodable texts are ones that contain a high number of words that use the sound-letter relationships that children are being taught as well as a limited number of high-frequency words." According to the National Reading Panel (2000), the benefit of this type of text is that it allows students to practice sequential decoding and develop the critical parts of beginning reading: fluency and automaticity. Cooper (2001) advised "even though decodable texts are most important in the beginning reading program, they may be needed in later grades for students who have not achieved independence in decoding" (p. 5).

More Word Families

After we read two or three chapters in Unit 1, I have my clients begin to see the word families. We have made up files for the J & J units and within each file are word family sticky notes. For Unit 1, for example, the –at and –am families are introduced through words such as cat, fat, sat, Sam, Tam, and am. Included among the many sorting activities corresponding to the J & J readers, *Sort It!* (Ferlito, 2000) includes word family sorts. I use the reproducible pages from this source or simply ask a child to sort the words printed on sticky notes into columns under –at or -am on the therapy table. For some reason, children have fun counting up which "family wins." Ferlito explained:

> Word sorting is a hands-on activity in which students arrange words according to specific attributes. This experience gives the students practice reading, comparing, and analyzing words, ultimately improving their reading and writing while engaging them in higher order thinking skills. (p. 3)

After some word sorting, I have the child copy and then print from memory the words and short phrases from the books we are reading onto the white board or paper. This is the perfect time to introduce any of the many word families/phonograms/phonic manipulatives that are available commercially or that you can make. One such source, *Fun Phonics Manipulatives* (Hancock, Pate, & Van-Haelst, 1997), is described by the authors as "phonetic pull-throughs." A 10- to 12-inch long strip of paper or file folder (about 1 inch wide) is cut to slide through another larger piece of paper or file folder that has a word family printed on it. As the 10- to 12-inch strip slides through the bigger piece, various consonants appear to help form words when placed in front of the word family printed on the bigger piece. This allows the child to see, become familiar with, and read various word families. The Hancock group (1997) described their manipulatives as follows:

> Each pull-through is shaped to represent one of the rhyming words in a group. For example, children make a dog-shaped pull-through for rhyming words with the *og* (family), starting with the word *dog*. As children begin to associate the rhyming blend with the picture, they can make the letter/sound link with words in other contexts (e.g., fog, hog, log, jog, frog). (p. 5)

As they get more experience with word families, it is helpful to add in some of the many word family materials available through publishing companies. I particularly like *Word Families and Silly Sentences* (2004). There are 75 silly sentence cards with illustrations and each sentence contains a number of examples of a particular word family. A few examples:

-ab family: A cr<u>ab</u> and a l<u>ab</u> rode in a c<u>ab</u>.

-amp family: The d<u>amp</u> c<u>amp</u> gave Dave a cr<u>amp</u>.

-at family: The f<u>at</u> c<u>at</u> wore a blue h<u>at</u>.

Word family charts can be purchased at teacher supply stores or downloaded at Web sites such as the one at http://carlscorner.us .com/Lists/Word%20Family%20

Web sites such as Jan Brett's include colorful phonograms/ word families: http://www.janbrett.com/phonograms/phonogram _at.htm

A number of "word family" books are available through publishers such as those included in the Learning Resources books. In these tiny books, a word family is introduced (e.g., -ap through words nap, snap, clap, and map). The pages that follow have short sentences (e.g., "Dad took a nap on the couch;" "Can you snap your fingers?" and "Clap your hands for the winner!)." See http://www.learning resources.com

Circling the Small Word Inside the Big Word

As soon the child is ready I teach him or her to begin to circle the small word inside the big word. So, even in the beginning words in the J & J readers, I have a child circle the -at inside "cat," and "sat" and "mat." The sooner children realize that big words are small words "glued together," the better equipped they become at decoding/word attack. I also like to download pages with word families and have children circle the word families within the printed words. Two sources include http://www.rhymezone.com and http://users .nac.net/dominica/wordfam.html

Making Big Words

Once a child understands that words are made up of smaller parts I introduce the notion of *making words* (Cunningham & Cunningham, 1992). You can download worksheets at http://classroom.jc-schools.net/read/Makewords.htm

In this technique, you print letters or give children letter tiles. You show them how to make words with the letters and then teach them to sort the words into word families So, for example, the letters [a b l s t] can make the words: at, lab, tab, sat, bat, bats, stab, last, and blast. These can be sorted as follows: -ab words: lab, tab; -at words: sat, bat, at; and -ast words: last, blast.

Rosner's (1987 and 1993) materials are beneficial here as well. By selecting the word family (referred to by Rosner as "Decoding Units"), you are reinforcing the idea that, when letters "stick together," they form word families. Photocopy the decoding unit (word family) pages you are working on from Rosner's books and have the child circle the family in as many words as s/he can. For example, the -ab family/decoding unit is included in monosyllabic words such as cab, dab, gab, slab, blab, drab; bisyllabic words such as shabby, blabber, cabin, habit, and multisyllabic words such as habitual, habitat, absolute. I do not have young children read these, only search with their eyes to find the printed word family.

More Writing to Expand Oral Language and Strengthen Reading and Writing

Once children are comfortable printing words, short phrases, and sentences from the J & J readers, or whatever early decoding material you are using, it is time to "pick back up" the strand of oral language. Now we encourage children to expand utterances through *oral and written language.* Two very strong sources I use for this include *Language! A Literacy Intervention Curriculum* (Eberhardt, Whitney, & Moats, 2000) and *Framing Your Thoughts* (Greene & Enfield, 1988). Although both of these resources work to expand written language, I have found them to be helpful in reinforcing and expanding oral language as well. In the Language Curriculum, a six-stage process is used to develop different sentence structures. The six stages are briefly described below:

Stage 1: Prepare Your Canvas: Base Subject + Base Predicate (e.g., "the birds flew")

Stage 2: Paint Your Predicate: through the addition of prepositional phrases or adverbs. The student is taught to add information to Stage 1 sentences through use of "how," "when," and "where" to Stage 1 sentences (e.g., "the birds flew fast", "the birds flew in the morning," and "the birds flew south")

Stage 3: Move the Predicate Painters: The student is now taught to move the predicate around in the sentence (e.g., "At night, the birds flew over the ocean")

Stage 4: Paint Your Subject: The student learns to describe the subject of the sentence through use of prepositional phrases, relative clause, and adjectives. She or he learns to mention "which," "what kind of," and "how many" to describe the subject (e.g., "the blue birds or fat birds or three birds flew . . . ")

Stage 5: Paint Your Words: The student is encouraged now to use more specific words to describe the words in the sentence (e.g., "the seagulls soared . . . "

Stage 6: Finishing Touches: The student is taught to move sentence parts around in the sentence (e.g., "at daybreak the fat, white seagulls soared . . . " or "the fat white seagulls soared at daybreak . . . "

Likewise, in *Framing Your Thoughts*, the student is taught about bare bone sentences; predicate word expansion using how, when, where, and why; use of prepositions; expanding the subject, connecting single words, parts of a sentence and sentences; garnishing a sentence, use of commas and ending punctuation. A strength of this program lies in its use of diagramming symbols. A sample of these includes: a straight line under the subject, a circle around the direct object, parentheses around the object of the preposition, and an up/down wiggly line under the predicate. The visual component adds much needed information in sentence expansion for most of the children with whom I work.

Keep Them Engaged in
Problem Solving, Creative Activities

Earlier, I mentioned the importance of knowing that the brain is a pattern seeker wanting to make sense of stimuli coming to it through all the senses. The focus of this resource has been on how to help children organize visual and auditory information to develop a stronger oral-written language system. The final section of this chapter offers suggestions to "keep kids engaged in problem-solving, creative activities" in a fun, not necessarily linguistic, way. I wish I had a penny for every time I've explained to the parents of many of my clients, "your child is so right-brained." In my experience, many children with language impairments, language-based reading, and writing problems love to engage in activities such as finding Waldo in the Where's Waldo books, or locating items in *I Spy* books. They like to build with Legos, and draw things, and manipulate jewelry, put together puzzles, move around, perhaps even dance. Unfortunately for them, learning much of our language is a left-brained activity as is learning to read and many other curricular activities at school. In his article "It Is Time to Get Serious About the Talents of Dyslexics," West (2008) cited Cohen's 1999 interview with William J, Dreyer, who was "a strong visual thinker and dyslexic . . . who developed new ways of thinking about molecular biology. . . . He (with his colleague, J. Claude Bennett) advanced a new theory and new data about genetics and the immune system that was 12 years ahead of everyone else in the field. They all had to learn to think the way he did" (p. 9).

Dreyer explained, "I knew I was different in the way that I thought, but I didn't realize why I was so dumb at spelling . . . and rote memory and arithmetic . . . " He describes an evening he and a colleague experienced when Dreyer told his colleague (both professors at Cal Tech in the Biology Division). "When I'm inventing an instrument or whatever, I see it in my head and I rotate it and try it out and move the gears. If it doesn't work, I rebuild it in my head" (p. 9).

In his book *In the Mind's Eye*, West (1997) held that,

> some of the most original thinkers in fields ranging from physical science and mathematics to politics and poetry have relied heavily on visual modes of thought . . . (yet) have shown evidence of a striking range of difficulties in their early schooling, including problems with reading, speaking, spelling, calculation, and memory. (p. 11)

Two terms I learned about some time ago I have found so aptly applies to our population of children: "learned helplessness" and "cognitive rigidity." It doesn't take too long for "our kids" to learn about how embarrassing it is to answer questions incorrectly or to misread words in front of peers in a classroom. It doesn't take too many of these painful experiences for our kids to start "shutting down" and responding verbally less and less of the time. They soon learn that others will answer the questions, that others will "bail them out" so they simply try less and less. They easily move into letting others answer for them and to quickly say "I don't know." They even learn that they don't have to say "I don't know" because people soon let them "get by" with shrugging their shoulders to nonverbally indicate "I don't know." The second term, cognitive rigidity, soon sets in. When our kids stop trying to answer the questions, they soon begin to think in certain rigid ways, they become less and less willing to take risks and become more and more rigid in the way they think about things. If you don't have your ideas challenged because you are not willing to take risks by talking about your ideas, you limit the expansion of your ability to cognitively navigate. We, as therapists, parents, and teachers, need to work steadfastly to increase our children's oral-written language skills. We also need to be mindful as to what our children's learning preference(s) are and build in activities that promote these as well.

Suggestions for Working on Problem Solving Creativity

I have no magic formula here, I just know that the children I have had the good fortune to work with over the years *love* it when they get to spend some part of their session with me engaged in some nonlinear, more right-brained activities. I always try to have the following items/games available in my therapy room:

Puzzles: a variety available from easy to more difficult. A little encouragement such as: "you can do it," "look for the edges," goes a long way.

Art work: drawing whatever they want on paper or the white board with many different colors. I also keep water colors, brushes, and paper in my room for my "budding artists."

Draw-And-Tell (Thompson, 1988) is a collection of stories intended to be used to increase a child's listening and narrative abilities. I like to use these to encourage a child to tell a story, for instance about "Alexander" which begins with "One day, Jesse took Alexander to the park. 'You wait here,' she said, 'I'm going to go and buy a balloon from the balloon man.' This is the balloon she bought." I draw a simple balloon (circle with a line coming down from it). I continue with the story drawing the parts ending up with the head of a teddy bear. After I read and draw two or three times, I ask the child to draw the items that will turn into something.

Games like "Rush Hour where the player has to manipulate objects such as plastic cars on a tray to allow a red car to pass. There are beginner, intermediate and advanced levels with a version on the computer at http://www.puzzles.com/products/RushHour.html

Divergent-Convergent Thinking

I debated as to whether I should include this discussion here or under oral language. I decided to put it here because it strongly supports encouraging a different kind of thinking. Convergent thinking refers to knowing specific details about something and "zeroing in on" or "converging" on the one correct answer. For example, we tell the child to think of something that is green and is round, and grows on trees and one correct answer would be "apple." Divergent thinking involves being given a specific answer and then the child elaborates ideas. Rather than one correct answer, there may be a number of possibilities. We change the above example to say: "Describe all the round, green things you can think of." This kind of mental activity is so useful in working with our population of children with language impairment because they tend to be such concrete thinkers. One of hundreds of examples comes to mind here. I am working with an 8-year-old boy with language impairment who loves to golf. He wanted to draw a golf club for me on the white board in my therapy room but alas! He said he could not do it. When I asked why not he explained "You don't have silver and black markers." We need to promote more flexible thinking!

Analogic Thinking

As in the above section, I pondered whether to include this section here or under oral language skills. And, as with divergent/convergent thinking, I decided to include it here for the same reasons. The Eides (Eide & Eide, 2005) explained: "Analogy is properly the domain of higher order thought because it requires fluency—lots of ideas —and integration across multiple representations. Analogy is also more simply thought of as flexible pattern recognition" (p. 1). Many resources exist to use in your work here and I'll mention just two. SuperDuper has produced *Analogies Fun Deck* (1998). A deck of cards has colorful drawings with printed words to help a child describe analogies, for instance: "hat is to head AS shoe is to _____"

Nelson and Gillespie's (1991) *Analogies for Thinking and Talking* is an entire volume of materials for working on analogies through words, pictures, and figures. These authors explained:

> Analogical reasoning, the ability to perceive similarities and differences between entities, is an important cognitive construct that emerges early in life and becomes increasingly refined during the course of an individual's development. At age 18 months, for example, the child who spontaneously calls a garden hose a 'snake' during symbolic play demonstrates a simple form of analogic reasoning. By age 18 years, however, the same person shows complex analogical reasoning in solving the following problem on a college entrance exam: *Heterogeneity is to divergence as homogeneity* is to _____. (p. i)

There are many other sources to increase problem solving and creative thinking. I invite the reader to not neglect this important part of working with children with oral-written language problems.

The purpose of this chapter was to provide an overview of how-tos to implement an oral-written language program for children in need of this development. To this end, seven key areas were selected for inclusion: oral language, phonological awareness, print awareness, alphabet knowledge, emergent writing, early reading and writing, and problem-solving/creative activities. The last two pages of this chapter (Figure 5–1) are included for practitioners to use in planning and implementing their sessions with children. They remind practitioners to move within and between the strands of oral-written language, thereby linking the strands of language and literacy. Remember to move around these strands mindful to "not get stuck" in any one of them. To help you with this a "language literacy strands goals and materials worksheet" has been included at the end of this chapter for you to duplicate and use as you work through the various strands. In addition to the strands covered in this chapter, the strands of Play and Listening Skills are listed on this worksheet.

The sixth and final chapter was written by Katie Lambert, MS, as a guide for using her accompanying CD to this resource. When

Katie was a graduate student in Speech-Language Pathology at California State University, Sacramento, she created a master's project that evolved into what she has put together for inclusion here. The focus of Chapter 6 and the CD is on two critical aspects discussed in this resource: oral narrative development and the need to use contextualized materials to strengthen children's developing language system.

LANGUAGE-LITERACY STRANDS TO INCLUDE IN MY THERAPY PLAN

TODAY'S DATE _____

FOR CLIENT _____

PLAY: yes/no

   GOAL: _____

   MATERIALS: _____

LISTENING SKILLS: yes/no

   GOAL: _____

   MATERIALS: _____

ORAL LANGUAGE: yes/no

   GOAL: _____

   MATERIALS: _____

PHONOLOGICAL AWARENESS: yes/no

   GOAL: _____

   MATERIALS: _____

Figure 5–1. *Sample Therapy Plan* continues

PRINT AWARENESS: yes/no

    GOAL: _____

    MATERIALS: _____

ALPHABET KNOWLEDGE: yes/no

    GOAL: _____

    MATERIALS: _____

EMERGENT WRITING:

    GOAL: _____

    MATERIALS: _____

EARLY READING & WRITING: yes/no

    GOAL: _____

    MATERIALS: _____

PROBLEM-SOLVING/CREATIVE ACTIVITIES: yes/no

    MATERIALS: _____

Figure 5–1. continued

Chapter 6

Oral Narration Outlines and Language Literacy Activities

Katie R. Lambert, MS, SLP

Introduction

Please refer to Chapter 5 of this resource for additional information on the importance of oral narrative skills in linking language and literacy.

For the purposes of this book, the authors have determined that using the story elements of character, setting, feelings (internal response), story starter (initiating event), stair step/transition words (episodes), and resolution to be adequate as a baseline for story-telling. The interventionist is encouraged to increase or decrease the story grammar per student's needs. In addition, the authors have chosen to incorporate writing elements containing Tier 1, basic words rarely requiring direct instruction for meaning, and Tier 2, high frequency words used across a variety of domains and important to the understanding of oral and written language (Beck, McKeown, & Kucan, 2002).

Interest in developing oral narrative skills in children has increased steadily over the past 20 years. Although authors vary as to terms and definitions, there is similarity among them as to what needs to be included in oral narratives. Table 6–1 summarizes five authors' work in this area.

Table 6–1. Elements of the Story

Story Grammar Model Stein & Glenn (1979)	Narrative Toolbox Hutson-Nechkash (2001)	Dynamic Assessment and Intervention Miller, Gillam, & Pena (2001)	Story Grammar Marker Moreau-Rooney & Fidrych (2002)	Test of Narrative Language Gillam & Pearson (2004)
Setting: introduces the characters, the location, and the time of the events	**Setting:** character, place, time	**Setting:** references to where and when the story occurs **Character information:** description of the characters	**Character:** who is the story about **Setting:** where does the story happen	**Macrostructure:** follows Stein and Glenn's (1979) Story Grammar Model **Setting:** introduces the characters, the location, and the time of the events
Initiating event: an action or happening that sets up a problem or dilemma for the story	**Problem:** first event, response, goal, plan, attempt	**Temporal order of events:** the sequencing of action **Causal relationships:** information about why the events occur	**Initiating event:** what happens to the character to cause them to do something	**Initiating event:** an action or happening that sets up a problem or dilemma for the story
Internal response: the main character's reaction to the initiating event			**Internal response:** how the character feels about the initiating event	**Internal response:** the main character's reaction to the initiating event

Story Grammar Model	Narrative Toolbox	Dynamic Assessment and Intervention	Story Grammar Marker	Test of Narrative Language
Internal plan: a statement of the goal; directed actions that the main character is thinking about taking; actions taken are called attempts			**Plan:** what the character will do; the most important element of Story Grammar Marker	**Internal plan:** a statement of the goal; directed actions that the main character is thinking about taking; actions taken are called attempts
Attempt: an action or plan of the character to solve the problem			**Attempt(s):** how does the character try to solve the problem(s); could be multiple attempts	**Attempt:** an action or plan of the character to solve the problem
Consequence: the result of the character's actions	**Solution:** outcome and ending		**Direct consequence:** what happened because of the attempt(s)	**Consequence:** the result of the character's actions
Reaction: a response by the character to the consequence			**Resolution:** how does the character feel about the consequence	**Reaction:** a response by the character to the consequence

continues

Table 6–1. *continued*

Story Grammar Model	Narrative Toolbox	Dynamic Assessment and Intervention	Story Grammar Marker	Test of Narrative Language
Ending: the conclusion of the story			**Critical thinking triangle:** used to answer the "why" questions from a story	**Ending:** the conclusion of the story
Episodes can be complete or incomplete. A complete episode must contain a minimum of these three elements: An initiating event or an internal response, an attempt and a direct consequence		**Story ideas and language:** *Complexity of idea*: the extent to which concepts are interconnected; *Complexity of vocabulary*: the extent to which vocabulary conveys nuances in meaning; *Grammatical complexity*: the degree of variation and complexity of the sentences in the story;	Has *developmental stages* for teaching preschool through adolescent.	**Microstructure:** proper nouns, action verbs, mental state verbs, temporal adverbs and casual adverbs. Syntax is more complex with more various and vocabulary that is more literature based.

Story Grammar Model	Narrative Toolbox	Dynamic Assessment and Intervention	Story Grammar Marker	Test of Narrative Language
		Knowledge of dialogue: the inclusion of spoken interaction between characters;	*Developmental checklist* begins a *descriptive sequence* (character and setting) and gradually builds to a *complex episode* (all items) and an *interactive episode* (all items and discusses a character's actions based on the actions of another character and answers the "why" questions of a story using the critical thinking triangle	
		Creativity: use of humor, irony, surprise, or mystery to make stories interesting and to captivate listeners' attention.		
		Episode structure:		
		Basic: includes an initiating event, or more attempts and a consequence	Use of a *hands on manipulative* to assist in anchoring the story sequence with students	
		Complete: elements of basic episode and internal response, plan and reaction/ending		
		Multiple: two or more complete and/or basic episodes		

How to Use These Materials

These materials and suggested uses for them have been found highly successful with the language-learning delayed/disabled students on my caseload as a speech and language pathologist. Materials are presented on the accompanying CD in the way I use them in my sessions.

What Oral Narration Level Is the Student?

First, you must decide if the student has enough knowledge of oral narration to begin retelling stories or if she or he requires additional support in the language of literacy (*characters, setting, problem, solution, plan, transition words*, etc.). If your student is ready to begin the storyboards, move onto storyboards; however, if she or he is struggling with the language of literacy, begin with preteaching sessions that increase both the understanding and use of this language.

Preteaching the Language of Literacy

When students with language-learning delays are given a storybook and told, "Tell me the story," most have a confused look as if to say, "What are you asking me to do?" or "Why do I need to tell it to you when you just read it?" For students who have language-learning delays, the language of literacy is yet another "foreign language" they must master to survive in the classroom. Simply asking them to state the characters, setting, problem and solution without giving an explanation as to what these words mean, adds to their confusion and frustration about language. This section includes several suggestions to help students comprehend and use the language of literacy.

Story Talk

Teaching students how to tell a story using the language of literacy can be challenging. However, given a label such as "story talk" for this special language facilitates students' learning and retaining the information with a higher success rate. Most of the time, for example, students can understand that a person is WHO the story is about, or a house is a PLACE or WHERE the story happens, but often they forget to use words such as character, setting, and so forth, especially if they are not exposed to it or have trouble learning the vocabulary. An example of a dialogue between an interventionist and child would be:

I(nterventionist): This is a picture of a _____

S(tudent): BOY!

I: Nice work! This is a boy! And what do we call a boy in Story Talk?

S: A person?

I: Yes, a boy is a person, but in Story Talk what do we call a person?

S: A character!

I: You are right! You're using your Story Talk!

Use of the term "Story Talk" sounds magical and fun, and it encourages the students to experiment with the language of literacy on a more consistent level. When introducing the language of literacy, remember to discuss Story Talk to provide a more concrete anchor for the student to remember the words.

Character(s)

What is a character? A character typically is a person or an animal and generally something that is alive with feelings. Be sure to emphasize that a character must have feelings, as this is important when discussing how the characters feel during story retell. By explaining to students that a character is a person or animal, you can begin making lists of people and animals.

Two examples of books that can be used to further illustrate the concept of "character" are *The Hat* (Brett, 1997) and *Stone Soup* (any version). In *The Hat*, the main character, Hedgie, talks with several different animals and one girl. *Stone Soup* includes several human characters including three soldiers, the villagers, and a mayor. Here are more ideas for preteaching characters:

- Use pictures of various items (animals, people, cars, food, etc.) and have students separate them into piles of what a character could and could not be.
- Hang up a large piece of paper in the room. Have the students list all the characters in the stories you read and tell whether they were animals or people.

Setting(s)

What is a setting? Simply put, the setting is a place. Do not engage with "it is where the story happens" yet. Let the student fully understand that a setting is a place, any place, before introducing a specific setting in a story. Just as you made lists for characters, make a separate list for settings (places). Have the student list as many places that she or he can recall. If they get stuck and cannot think of more, give them hints such as, "Where do you like to go on the weekends?" or "Where is your favorite place to go on vacation?" Usually they know of more places but require prompts to help them realize and verbalize it. Once they have fully grasped the concept of what a place is, introduce that in a story, the place where the story happens is called the setting. Sample books for additional teaching of the concept of setting, include: *We're Going on a Bear Hunt* (Rosen, 1989) where a family goes through many different places on their hunt for a bear and *Corduroy* (Freeman, 1968) where a teddy bear lives in a department store.

Additional ideas for preteaching settings:

- Use pictures of various items and have the students separate them into piles of places and pictures that are not places.
- Hang up a large piece of paper in the room. Whenever you read a book have the student list the place where the story happened (could be more than one place; now is the time to start using the word setting).

Problem(S)

What is a problem? Most students will understand what a "problem" is, but may not link the word "problem" to specific situations. They may understand that something is not right or that something needs to be fixed, but not that it is called a *problem*. One of the simplest ways to teach the word "problem" is to set up a demonstration where something goes wrong. For instance, during an art project forget the scissors and ask, "How are we going to cut the paper?" Spill a box of items on the floor and say, "We've got a mess on the floor. Now that's a problem." Whenever something does not work out the way it should, use the word "problem." This way the students are connecting the word to the situations and emotions. Keep in mind that a problem is not always a bad thing; sometimes it is simply that something needs to be accomplished, but one cannot think of a way to accomplish it. One of the best books to help teach the concept "problem" is *That's Good! That's Bad!* (Cuyler, 1991). In this short story, a little boy is carried off by a balloon and endures various obstacles; some are good and some are bad. When reading this story, ask the students what the problem is on each page. Additionally, hang up a large piece of paper in the room, draw a line down the middle, and separate the paper in to *Problem, Solution*. After reading a story, have the children list the problem(s) under the problem side of the paper. After they have learned about solutions, they can go back and fill in the solutions to the problems.

Solution(s)

What is a solution? A solution is how to solve (or fix) the problem. Since students have previously learned what a "problem" is, have them state how they would then solve (or fix) those problems. *Maisy Makes Lemonade* (Cousins, 2002) is great for illustrating the concept of solutions. In this story, the main character, Maisy, solves the problem of running out of lemonade by making more lemonade. *The Little Red Hen* (any version) also provides an example of a solution when the little red hen does all the work by herself when her lazy friends will not help.

Story Starter(s)

The discussion of story starters is divided into three sections: Beginning Storytellers, Intermediate Storytellers, and Advanced Storytellers.

When teaching beginning storytellers (developing pre-kindergarten/kindergarten) who struggle with starting a story, provide them the formula of *When* (represented by a clock) + *Who* (a stick figure) + *Where* (a house) + *Do* (write the word). This formula is provided in icons on the accompanying CD. The steps for accomplishing this are as follows:

1. Ask the students **when** the story happened: "Once upon a time," "One day," "Today," etc.
2. **Who** is in the story: looking for the character names
3. **Where** is the story happening: looking for the setting
4. What does the character(s) want to **do**?: "pick blueberries" (*Blueberries for Sal*), "eat food" (*The Very Hungry Caterpillar*), "find his button" (*Corduroy*)

An example of a beginning story starter for *Blueberries for Sal* would be:

One day, Little Sal and her mom wanted to make blueberry jam, but they did not have any blueberries. So, they went to Blueberry Hill to pick some blueberries. Little Sal and her mom were excited to pick blueberries for blueberry jam.

Intermediate storytellers (developmentally lower elementary) should be encouraged to begin a story with any opening they want. *Note:* they should have been exposed to the various story openers and transition words (see later section) by this point. After the opener, they need to state the problem, solution, the plan to accomplish the solution, and how the characters felt about it.

Advanced storytellers should be given freedom to create their own story starters as long as it stays with the same basic story sequence.

There are several books available with a variety of story starters; some examples are:

- *The Very Hungry Caterpillar* (Carle, 1987)
  "In the light of the moon a little egg lay on a leaf."

- *Happy Birthday, Moon* (Asch, 1982)
  "One night Bear looked up at the sky and thought, wouldn't it be nice to give the moon a birthday present."

- *The Very Quiet Cricket* (Carle, 1990)
  "One warm day, from a tiny egg a little cricket was born."

- *The Mitten* (adapted, Brett, 1989)
  "Once there was a boy named Nicki who wanted his new mittens made from wool as white as snow."

Most fairytales begin with wonderful story starters; "Once upon a time . . . ," "One time in faraway land . . . ," "Many years ago not so far away . . . ," and so forth.

When reading with your students, emphasize the story starters and see who can notice the different types. Keep a list of these as they will be beneficial when the students begin writing their own stories.

Feelings/How Did They Feel About That?

When introducing what a "character" is (person or animal), emphasize to students that characters have feelings. For most students, feelings come naturally. Everyone has feelings, but not everyone knows the words that go with the feelings they are having. A favorite way to teach feelings is to have a feelings contest. If working with a student individually, sit with your student side by side and face a mirror so that you both can see each other's faces in the mirror. Using either picture cards depicting emotions or written emotions (depending on the level of the student) take turns pantomiming that emotion in the mirror while the other guesses the emotion (happy, sad, mad, worried, etc.). If in a group setting, each student has a chance to pantomime the emotions while the rest of the group guesses at the emotions.

Reading books that illustrate characters with exaggerated emotions helps in matching words with feelings/emotions. *Parts*

(Arnold, 1997) shows a little boy with wonderful emotions and students will love discovering his emotions (worried, scared, happy, etc.).

Pigs Can't Fly (Cort, 2002) and *Corduroy* (Freeman, 1968) explicitly state how the characters feel:

> "I'm bored. Bored, bored, bored, bored, bored!"
> (*Pigs Can't Fly*)

> "Corduroy watched them sadly as they walked away"
> (*Corduroy*)

As with other Story Talk concepts, keep a list of feelings that the various characters experience.

Stairstep Words (Transition Words)

Stairstep words are the transition words needed to move between events (or episodes) within a story. Words such as *first, next, then,* and *finally* are all considered stairstep words. They are called stairstep words because students are taught that a story has a sequence of steps and in telling about the steps we "climb up the stairs." This is a good visual for students and tends to stay with them better than simply telling them to say *first, next, then,* and so forth. Some ways to teach stairstep words are:

- Print out several pictures of stairs and put them in a row on the table or floor. After reading a story, talk about the events in the story and walk up the stairs while saying, "First, next, then, and so forth."
- Cut out brown or gray construction paper to look like pathway stones and lay them on the ground. After reading a story, have students walk across each stone as they talk about each event in the story using the Stairstep Words.
- Cut out construction paper to look like lily pads. Use the same general instructions as the pathway stones, but they can jump like frogs from lily pad to lily pad.

Using Storyboards, Outlines, and Additional Materials

Storyboards

The storyboards included with these materials are divided into four levels: preschool, beginning, intermediate, and advanced. It is important to first identify students' levels of oral narrations and which storyboard is developmentally appropriate. In other words, preschoolers/kindergartners should not be using the advanced storyboards, nor lower elementary students working on preschool or beginning storyboards, unless they need the basics of storytelling prior to working at their developmentally appropriate level. The interventionist will be required to download pictures from the storybook, clipart, or other image software for each storyboard. Suggested icons are provided on individual storyboards.

The interventionist will be required to download pictures from the storybook, clipart, or other image software for each storyboard. Provided on the accompanying CD are two versions of the beginning storyboards: PDF files and individual Word documents. Interventionists choosing to print, cut, and glue icons to the storyboards should use the PDF files, whereas interventionists preferring to download icons directly to the storyboards should use the Word document version.

Before beginning the storyboards, it is suggested that a book be read at least three times to the student. It has been found most successful to follow these steps when reading the book with the student:

- *First time:* Read the story to the student and point out how the pictures in the book are helping to tell the story.
- *Second time:* Read the story with the student and ask Wh-questions. It has been found that Wh-questions build additional comprehension of the story and that the students will add this additional information in their storytelling.
- *Third time:* Have the student "read" the story by looking at the pictures and using his or her Story Talk. If they leave out any important information, ask them a Wh- question. The student can "read" the story more than once. When you feel they have a solid understanding of the story, move them onto the storyboard.

Preschool

Preschool storyboards involve retelling the story with icons printed from clipart, the books, or other picture software. Cut out the icons and glue them to sticky notes. Have the student practice putting the images in the order of what happened in the book. Do a simple version of the story, encouraging the student to use his or her Story Talk. You may need to model or prompt the Story Talk for students as they have just learned the pieces and are now being asked to put all the pieces together to create a story. Another activity for preschoolers is to cut out stepping stones or lily pads from construction paper, lay them on the ground and have the students jump from one lily pad or stepping stone for each event in the story. Each time the student jumps, they need to use a stairstep word (*first, next, then, finally*, etc.).

Beginning

Remember to download pictures from the storybook, clipart, or other image software for each storyboard. Suggested images are provided on individual storyboards.

Once the students successfully retell the stories at the preschool level, they can move to the beginning storyboard, where they are instructed to retell the story by using icons representing the story. It is important for the student to have an understanding of the story before moving on to the beginning storyboard to increase successful retell.

Beginning storyboards move left to right, top to bottom, starting with the first character name all of the characters. Move down and left, then state the setting, story starter and the character(s) feelings. Now move down and left, and begin telling the story (using Story Talk) using the icons and ending on the "finally" icon. Once the student can independently retell the story using the beginning storyboard, move to intermediate/advanced storyboards only if this is developmentally appropriate. If it is not developmentally appropriate, continue with beginning storyboards diminishing the amount of visual and verbal prompts.

Intermediate/Advanced

The intermediate and advanced storyteller should be encouraged to retell the story at this level using generic rather than specific icons used in beginning storyboards, but their storytelling will be different. This outline does not require the interventionist to download images; the generic images provided will suffice for these levels of oral narratives.

The intermediate storyteller will use a variety of story starters and transition words while telling the story. They also will follow an outline that does not give clues to the flow of the story through "specific icons"; rather "generic icons" and students must recall the story in order to retell it.

Advanced

Advanced storytellers are given full freedom to create their own story. It is important to note that advanced storytellers are not retelling a story previously read, but are creating an original story.

Using the same outline from the intermediate level, have the students brainstorm characters, setting, story starter, problem, solution, feelings, and steps in the story. If they cannot come up with an idea for a story, you may need to prompt them; usually a personal narrative is easier than fictional narratives. Write the ideas on a whiteboard, making each part of the story color-coded (character names = green, setting = yellow, problem = blue, etc.), which helps the students keep the story in order. After the story has been brainstormed and written on the whiteboard, the students copy the information to their outline and verbally tell their story.

There are basic story outlines located at the end of the materials located on the accompanying CD. These outlines are intended as quick references for the interventionist as the student(s) are using the beginning and intermediate storyboards

Writing

I have found that when students practice listening, saying, and writing about materials being taught the information and skills are understood, retained, and retrieved at a more automatic and accurate level.

Beginning Writing

Students who are at the beginning stage of storytelling should be given the beginning writing pages. There are two levels of writing for the beginning writer.

First level: Download images from clipart, the storybooks, or other picture software into the provided templates; the pictures should be simple enough for the students to attempt to copy. The students are instructed to copy the picture the best they can in the empty boxes. Two pages per book have been provided along with a blank template for additional drawing. The students can copy pictures from the book or even the alphabet and numbers depending on their level.

Second level: Each page contains individual Tier 1 and Tier 2 words, and the student is instructed to copy the words into the blank boxes.

Intermediate Writing

Students at the intermediate level of storytelling should be given the intermediate writing tasks. However, it should be taken into consideration that if the student's oral language skills are higher than his or her written language skills keep him or her at the lower level until proficient before moving to more advanced levels of writing. There are two levels of writing for the intermediate writer.

First level: The student is given a page containing short sentences from the storybook, which she or he directly copies onto the blank lines. Since these sentences come from the storybook, they will contain Tier 2 vocabulary words.

Second level: The student is given a page containing cloze sentences. The student chooses a word from a word bank in order to complete the sentences. These sentences are from stories and contain Tier 1 and Tier 2 vocabulary words.

Advanced Writing

There are multiple activities that can be used at this level.

- *Activity 1:* The student verbally states a sentence while the interventionist writes it on the whiteboard, the student then copies the sentences onto their writing paper.

- *Activity 2:* The student orally narrates a story as the interventionist writes the outline on a whiteboard. The student then copies the outline on the whiteboard to their paper outline.
- *Activity 3:* The student fills out his or her own outline independently.
- *Activity 4:* The student fills out the paper outline and then copies it to writing paper in a story form. Make sure they give their masterpiece a title and draw a picture to go with it.

These activities are more effective if used in progression and not simultaneously.

Wh-Questions

As stated earlier, Wh-questions help to increase both receptive and expressive language skills. The various activities for Wh-questions are:

- Ask the wh- questions while reading the stories. A sample page of questions is provided on the accompanying CD.
- Using the paper dice template, located on the accompanying CD, write the words "What," "Who," "Where," "When," "Why," and "How" on different sides of the dice. Have the student roll the dice and answer the type of question he or she rolls. This is a wonderful tool as it makes the students feel in control of their learning. This can be switched so that they have to come up with the type of question they rolled to ask you.
- The paper dice questions can be used to ask or answer questions about the story or about anything in general (the therapy room, the student's weekend, favorite toys/games, etc.). Be creative!

Extras

Included in the accompanying CD are a few extra materials for the interventionist to use with students. There are suggestions for using these materials; however, the interventionist is strongly encouraged to tap into their imagination and be creative with these materials in order to use them successfully.

Paper Dice

- Write Story Talk words including character, setting, and so forth, in the blank spaces and have the students roll the dice and give the answer for the current story you are working on or the story they have written. This also can be used to help the student(s) brainstorm for an advanced story.
- Glue on various pictures and ask the student(s) to tell if the picture is a character, setting, problem, solution, and so on.
- Glue on various pictures depicting problems and have the student(s) tell what the problem(s) in the pictures are and how they might solve them.

Personal Storytelling Binder/Notebook/Journal

Provide a notebook, three-ring binder, or folder for each student to keep storytelling materials.

Included on the accompanying CD are Story Talk pages for each of the 12 books used on the CD. Each page has all of the elements of storytelling that have been taught over the course of this section.

After reading a storybook, provide the student with a copy of the Story Talk page. The student will fill in the Story Talk page as she or he learns each element. If she or he is in the more advanced stages of storytelling, he or she can fill out the information as they think of it and turn it in as an assignment.

Pocket Chart Pictures

Provided on the accompanying CD are pocket chart pictures representing each element of Story Talk. There are a few different ways you can use these pictures to further cement oral narratives. The following suggestions are how I have used them in my sessions, however, the interventionist is encouraged to use them however he or she needs to facilitate Story Talk.

- Put the Story Talk icons into the pocket chart and provide the student with pictures representing each story element specific to the book used. Have the student place the picture next to the correct Story Talk icon. For example, if working with the book *The Hat* (Brett, 1997), give the student all the animal pictures representing the characters, a farm representing the setting, a sad face representing how Hedgie felt, and so forth. The student then places the animal pictures next to the character icon, the farm next to the setting icon and the sad face next to the heart icon.
- Begin retelling the story with the student placing the correct pictures in the pocket chart. This is a great activity for groups as well as individual students.
- Use the paper dice (discussed above) in conjunction with the pocket chart; instruct the student to roll the dice containing elements of Story Talk. Whichever element the student rolls he or she must find the correct picture and place it next to the correct icon.

It is my sincerest hope that through this supplemental CD and the activities shared, as an interventionist you will tap into your creative and imaginative side and begin to expand on these activities as you see fit for your students.

References

Ahlberg, J., & Albert, A. (1995). *The jolly pocket postman or other people's letters.* London, UK: William Heinemann Ltd.

American Speech-Language-Hearing Association. (2001). *Roles and responsibilities of speech-language pathologists with respect to reading and writing in children and adolescents.* Washington, DC: Author.

American Speech-Language-Hearing Association, Working Group on Auditory Processing Disorders. (2005). *(Central) auditory processing disorders.* [Technical report]. Rockville, MD: Author.

Analogies fun deck (1998). Greenville, SC: SuperDuper.

Anderson, N. A. (2006). *Elementary children's literature: The basics for teachers and parents.* Boston, MA: Allyn & Bacon.

Anglin, J. M. (1993). Vocabulary development: A morphological analysis. *Monographs of the Society for Research in Child Development, 10*(238), 1–166.

Arnold, T. (1997). *Parts.* New York, NY: Penguin Books USA.

Asch, F. (1982). *Happy birthday, moon.* New York, NY: Aladdin Paperbacks.

Baddeley, A., Gathercole, S., & Papagno, C. (1988). The phonological loop as a language learning device. *Psychological Review, 105*(1), 158–173.

Bailer, K. (2003). *Developmental stages of scribbling.* Retrieved June 2009, from http://www.k-play.com

Ball, S. (1985a). *Crocuphant.* Bridgeport, CT: WJ Fantasy.

Ball, S. (1985b). *Porguacan.* Bridgeport, CT: WJ Fantasy.

Banks, K. (1988). *Alphabet soup.* New York, NY: Alfred A. Knopf.

Base, G. (1986). *Anamalia.* New York, NY: Harry N. Abrams.

Beaty, J. J. (2008). *50 early childhood literacy strategies.* Boston, MA: Allyn & Bacon. Retrieved September 21, 2009, from http://www.education.com/reference/article/early-writing-scribbling/

Beck, I., McKeown, M., & Kucan, L. (2002). *Bringing words to life—robust vocabulary instruction.* New York, NY: Guilford Press.

Bellis, T. J. (2001, (April). *Assessment and management of auditory processing disorders.* Presentation at California Speech-Language-Hearing Association Annual State Conference. Monterey, CA.

Bellis, T. J. (2003). *Assessment and management of central auditory processing disorders in the education setting* (2nd ed.). Clifton Park, NY: Thomson Delmar Learning.

Benson, D. F. (1994). *The neurology of thinking.* New York, NY: Oxford University Press.

Bishop, D. V. M., & Edmundson, A. (1987). Language impaired four year olds: Distinguishing transient from persistent impairment. *Journal of Speech and Hearing Disorders, 52,* 156–173.

Blockcolsky, V.D., Frazer, J. M., & Frazer, D. H. (1987). *40,000 selected words: Organized by letter and sound.* Tuscon, AZ: Communication Skill Builders.

Boggle Junior Letters. (1992). Pawtucket, RI: Hasbro.

Brett, J. (1989). *The mitten: A Ukrainian folk tale.* New York, NY: G. P. Putnam's Sons.

Brett, J. (1997). *The Hat.* New York, NY: Scholastic.

Brown, H. D. (2007). *Principles of language learning and teaching* (5th ed.). Retrieved August 29, 2009, from http://languagelinks2006.wikispaces .com/Implicit+vs.+Explicit+Teaching

Brown, R. (1973). *A first language: The early stages.* Cambridge, MA: Harvard University Press.

Bruner, J. (1981). The social context of language acquisition. *Language and Communication, 1,* 155–178.

Burrows, R. (n.d.). *Word magic: Magnetic sentence builder.* Wayne, PA: Sandvik Innovations, LLC.

Butler, K. (1999). Foreword. *Topics in Language Disorders, 20,* iv–v.

Cabell, S. Q., Justice, L. M., Kaderavek, J. N., Turnbull, K. P., & Breit-Smith, A. (2009). *Emergent literacy: Lessons for success.* San Diego, CA: Plural Publishing.

California Language-Speech-Hearing Association. (2002). *Position paper on central auditory processing disorders.* Sacramento, CA: Author.

Capucilli, A. S. (1995). *Inside a barn in the country.* New York, NY: Scholastic.

Capucilli, A. S. (1998). *Inside a house that is haunted.* New York, NY: Scholastic.

Carey, S. (1978). The child as word learner. In M. Halle, J. Bresnan, & G. A. Miller (Eds.), *Linguistic theory and psychological reality.* Cambridge, MA: MIT Press.

Carle, E (1987). *The very hungry caterpillar.* New York, NY: Philomel Books.

Carle, E (1990). *The very quiet cricket.* New York, NY: Philomel Books.

Carle, E. (1998). *The secret birthday message.* New York, NY: Harper-Collins.

Catts, H., & Kamhi, A. (2005). Causes of reading disabilities. In H. Catts & A. Kamhi (Eds.), *Language and reading disabilities* (2nd ed., pp. 94-126). Boston, MA: Allyn & Bacon.

Chomsky, N. (1980). *Rules and representations.* New York, NY: Columbia University Press.

Clements. A. (1997). *Double trouble in walla walla.* Brookfield, CT: Millbrook Press.

Cole, K. N., Maddox, M. E., & Lim, Y. S. (2006). Language is the key: Constructive interactions around books and play. In R. J. McCauley & M. E. Frey (Eds.), *Treatment of language disorders in children* (pp. 149-174). Baltimore, MD: Paul H. Brookes.

Colorado, C. (2008). *Helping young children develop strong writing skills.* Retrieved June, 2009, from http://www.colorincolarado.org/article/21885

Cooper, J. D. (2001). *Using different types of texts for effective reading instruction.* Retrieved August 15, 2009 from www.eduplace.com/state/author/jdcooper.pdf

Cort, B (2002). *Pigs can't fly.* New York, NY: Barron's Grosset Book Group.

Cousins, L. (1999). *Maisy's bedtime.* Cambridge, MA: Candlewick Press.

Cousins, L. (2000). *Maisy's drives a bus.* Cambridge, MA: Candlewick Press.

Cousins, L. (2001). *Maisy goes shopping.* Cambridge, MA: Candlewick Press.

Cousins, L. (2002). *Maisy makes lemonade.* Cambridge, MA: Candlewick Press.

Cunningham, P. M., & Cunningham, J. W. (1992). Making words: Enhancing the invented spelling-decoding connection. *Reading Teacher, 46,* 106-115.

Curious George: Reading and phonics [Software]. (2002), New York, NY: Houghton-Mifflin.

Cuyler, M (1991). *That's good, That's bad!* New York, NY: Henry Holt and Company

Damico, J. S. (1988). The lack of efficacy in language therapy: A case study. *Language, Speech and Hearing Services in Schools, 19,* 51-66.

Davis, L. (1994). *P. B. bear's birthday party.* London, UK: Kindersley Ltd.

Degen, B. (1983). *Jamberry.* New York, NY: HarperCollins.

Dickinson, D., & McCabe, A. (1991). The acquisition and development of language: A social interactionist account of language and literacy development. In J. F. Kavanagh (Ed.), *The language continuum: From infancy to literacy* (pp. 1-40). Parkton, MD: York Press.

Earobics. (1997, 1998). http://www.earobics.com

Eberhardt, N. C., Whitney, A., & Moats, L. C. (2000). *Language! A literacy intervention curriculum.* Longmont, CO; Sopris West.

Edwards. B. (1999). *The new drawing on the right side of the brain.* New York, NY: Tarcher/Putnam.

Eide, B., & Eide, F. (2005). *The power of analogical thinking.* Retrieved September 5, 2009, from http://eideneurolearningblog.blogspot.com/2005

Ferlito, S. (2000). *Sort it! Word sorting activities to complement the language! curriculum.* Longmont, CO: Sopris West.

Fernie, D. (2000). *The nature of children's play.* Retrieved May, 2009, from http://www.kidsource/content2/Nature.of.Child's.play.html

Ferre, J. M. (2007). The ABCs of CAP: Practical strategies for enhancing central auditory processing skills. In D. S. Geffner & D. Ross-Swain (Eds.), *Auditory processing disorders: Assessment, management, and treatment* (pp. 187–206). San Diego, CA: Plural Publishing.

Fey, M. (1986). *Language intervention with young children.* San Diego, CA: College-Hill Press.

Freeman, D (1968). *Corduroy.* New York, NY: Viking Press.

Gebers, J. (2003). *Books are for talking too! A sourcebook for using children's literature in speech-language remediation.* Tucson, AZ: Communication Skill Builders.

Geffner, D. S. (2007). Central auditory processing disorders: Definition, description, and behaviors. In D. S. Geffner & D. Ross-Swain (Eds.), *Auditory processing disorders: Assessment, management, and treatment* (pp. 25–47). San Diego, CA: Plural Publishing.

Geffner, D. S., & Ross-Swain, D. (Eds.). (2007). *Auditory processing disorders: Assessment, management, and treatment* (pp. 3–24). San Diego, CA: Plural Publishing.

Geisel, T. S., & Geisel, A. S. (1957). *Cat in the hat by Dr. Seuss.* New York, NY: Beginner Books, A division of Random House.

Gillam, R. B., & Pearson N. A. (2004). *Test of narrative language.* Austin, TX: Pro-Ed.

Gillet, P. (1993). *Auditory processes.* Novato, CA: Academic Therapy Publications.

Gillon, G. (2004). *Phonological awareness: From research to practice.* New York, NY: Guilford Press.

Girolametto, L., & Weitzman, E. (2006). It takes two to talk-The Hanen program for parents: Early language intervention through caregiver training. In R. J. McCauley & M. E. Frey (Eds.), *Treatment of language disorders in children* (pp. 77–104). Baltimore, MD: Paul H. Brookes.

Gitlin-Weiner, K., Sandarund, A., & Schaefer, C. (Eds.). *Play diagnosis and assessment* (pp.15–57). New York, NY: Wiley.

Go Fish for Letters. (1996). Burlingame, CA: University Games Corporation.

Goldone, P. (1973). *The little red hen.* New York, NY: Clarion Books.

Goldsworthy, C. (1998). *Sourcebook of phonological awareness training: Children's classic literature* (Vol. 2). San Diego, CA: Singular Publishing Group.

Goldsworthy, C. (2000). *Sourcebook of phonological awareness training: Children's core literature.* San Diego, CA: Singular Publishing Group.

Goldsworthy, C. (2003). *Developmental reading disabilities: A language based reading program.* Clifton Park, NY: Singular/Delmar-Thomson.

Goldsworthy, C., & Pieretti, R. (2004*). Sourcebook of phonological awareness training: Children's core literature* (Vol. 3). Clifton Park, NY: Delmar Thomson Learning .

Greene, V. E., & Enfield, M. L. (1988). *Framing your thoughts: The basic structure of written expression.* Bloomington, MN: Language Circle Enterprise.

Greene, V. E., & Woods, J. F. (2000). *J & J language readers.* Longmont, CO: Sopris West.

Greenspan, S., & Weider, S. (1998). *The child with special needs: Encouraging intellectual and emotional growth.* New York, NY: Perseus Books.

Grossen, B. (1997). *A synthesis of research on reading from the National Institute of Child Health and Human Development.* Retrieved June 2000, from http://www.nrrf.org/synthesis_research.htm

Hamaguchi, P., & Tazeau, Y. N. (2007). Comorbidity of APD with other "look-alikes." In D. S. Geffner & D. Ross-Swain (Eds.), *Auditory processing disorders: Assessment, management, and treatment* (pp. 49–74). San Diego, CA: Plural Publishing.

Hancock, M., Pate, S., & VanHaelst, J. (1997). *Fun phonics manipulatives.* New York, NY: Scholastic Professional Books.

Hanford, M. (n.d.). *Where's Waldo Series.* Cambridge, MA: Candlewick Press.

Hart, B., & Risley, T. R. (1995). *Meaningful differences in the everyday experiences of young American children.* Baltimore, MD: Paul H. Brookes.

Hawkins, C. & J. (1987). *I know an old lady who swallowed a fly.* New York, NY: G. P. Putnam's Sons.

Hegde, M. N., & Pomaville, F. (2008). *Assessment of communication disorders in children: Resources and protocols.* San Diego, CA: Plural Publishing.

Highlights Magazine. Columbus, OH: Highlights.

Hill, E. (1980). *Where's Spot?* London, UK: Ventura Publishing Ltd.

Hodson, B., & Paden, E. (1991). *Targeting intelligible speech: A phonological approach to remediation* (2nd ed.). Austin, TX: Pro-Ed.

Hubbell, R. D. (1996). Facilitative play. Personal communication.

Hutson-Nechkash, P. (2001). *Narrative toolbox: Blueprints for story building success.* Eau Claire, WI: Thinking Publications.

I spy books (e.g., *I spy school days* [1995], and *I spy treasure hunt* [1999]). Photographs by Walter Wick and Riddles by Jean Marzollo. New York: NY: Scholastic.

Johnson, C. J., & Yeates, E. (2006). *Evidence-based vocabulary instruction for elementary students via storybook reading. EPB Brief* (Vol 1, No. 3). Upper Saddle River, NJ: Pearson Education.

Johnston, J. (2006). *Thinking about child language: Research to practice.* Eau Claire, WI: Thinking Publications.

Justice, L. M. (2007, August). *Evidence-based intervention: Approaches for emergent literacy.* Presentation at Leading Best Practices in Language and Literacy Conference, Monterey, CA.

Justice, L. M., & Ezell, H. K. (2001). Word and print awareness in 4-year-old children. *Child Language Teaching and Therapy, 17,* 207–225.

Justice, L. M., & Ezell, H. K. (2004). Print referencing: An emergent literacy enhancement strategy and its clinical applications. *Language, Speech, and Hearing Services in Schools, 35,* 185–193.

Justice, L. M., & Kaderavek, J. (2004). Embedded-explicit emergent literacy intervention I: Background and description of approach, *Language, Speech, and Hearing Services in Schools, 35,* 201–211.

Justice, L. M., Meier, J., & Walpole, S. (2005). Learning new words from storybooks: An efficacy study with at-risk kindergartners. *Language, Speech, and Hearing Services in Schools, 36,* 17–32.

Kaderavek, J. N., & Justice, L. (2002). Shared storybook reading as an intervention context: Practices and potential pitfalls. *American Journal of Speech-Language Pathology, 11,* 395–406.

Keith, R. W. (2000). *RGDT: The Random Gap Detection Test.* St. Louis, MO: Auditec.

Kent, R. D. (1990). The fragmentation of clinical service and clinical science in communicative disorders. *National Student Speech Language Hearing Association Journal, 17,* 4–16.

Languagelinks. (2006). *Explicit vs. implicit teaching and learning.* Retrieved November 5, 2009, from http://www.Languagelinks2006 wikispaces.com/Implicit+vs.+Explicit+Teaching

Lee, L. (1974). *Developmental sentence analysis: A grammatical assessment procedure for speech and language clinicians.* Evanston, IL: Northwestern University Press.

Leonard, L. B, Eyer, J. A., Bedore, L. M., & Greta, B. G. (1997). Three accounts of the grammatical morpheme difficulties of English speaking children with specific language impairment. *Journal of Speech and Hearing Research, 40,* 741–753.

Lindamood, P., & Lindamood, P. (1998). *Lindamood phoneme sequencing program for reading, spelling, and speech* (3rd ed.). Austin, TX: Pro-Ed.

Locke, J. (1997). A theory of neurolinguistic development. *Brain and Language, 58*, 265-326.

Lovelace, S., & Stewart, S. R. (2007). Increasing print awareness in preschoolers with language impairment using non-evocative print referencing. *Language, Speech, and Hearing Services in Schools, 38*, 16-30.

Lowenfeld, V. (1987). *Creative and mental growth* (4th ed.). New York, NY: Macmillan.

Luker, J. R. (2007). History of auditory processing and its disorders in children. In D. S. Geffner & D. Ross-Swain (Eds.), *Auditory processing disorders: Assessment, management, and treatment* (pp. 3-24). San Diego, CA: Plural Publishing.

Lyon, G. R. (1997). "SLPs play key role," Seymour tells NIH conference on LD. *ASHA Leader, 2*, 1-5.

Martin, B., & Archambault, J. (1988). *Listen to the rain.* New York, NY: Henry Holt.

Martin, B., & Archambault, J. (2002). *Chicka chicka boom boom ABC magnet book.* New York, NY: Henry Holt.

Marvin, C. A., & Wright, D. (1997). Literacy socialization in the homes of preschool children. *Language, Speech, and Hearing Services in Schools, 28*, 154-163.

Mayer, M. (1969). *Frog, where are you?* New York, NY: Dial Books for Young Readers.

Mayer, M. (1971). *A boy, a dog, a frog, and a friend.* New York, NY: Dial Books for Young Readers.

Mayer, M. (1974). *Frog goes to dinner.* New York. NY: Dial Books for Young Readers.

Mayer, M. (1986). *There's an alligator under my bed.* New York, NY: Dial Books for Young Readers.

McCabe, A., & Rollins, P. R. (1992, March). *Assessment of preschool narrative skills: Prerequisite for literacy.* Presentation at the International Conference of the Learning Disabilities Association, Atlanta, GA.

McCauley, R. J., & Fey, M. E. (2006). *Treatment of language disorder in children.* Baltimore, MD: Paul H. Brookes.

McCloskey, R. (1949). *Blueberries for Sal.* New York, NY: The Viking Press.

Miller, L., Gillam, R. B., & Pena, E. D. (2001). *Dynamic assessment and intervention.* Austin, TX: Pro-Ed.

Mitton, T. (2002). *Dinosaurumpus.* New York, NY: Scholastic.

Moreau-Rooney, M., & Fidrych, H. (2002). *Story grammar marker* [Learning tool]. Springfield, MA: MindWing Concepts.

Mosel, A. (1968). *Tiki tiki tembo.* New York, NY: Scholastic.

Most, B. (1991). *Pets in trumpets: And other word-play riddles.* San Diego, CA: Harcourt Brace Jovanovich.

Nagy, W., & Anderson, R. (1984). The number of words in printed English. *Reading Research Quarterly, 19*, 304–330.

National Network for Child Care. (2009). Available from http://www.nncc.org/Curriculum/better.play.html

National Early Literacy Panel. (2004, November). *The National Early Literacy Panel: A research synthesis on early literacy development.* Presentation to the National Association of Early Childhood Specialists, Anaheim, CA.

National Institutes of Health. (2004). *Central auditory processing disorder* (Pub. No. 01-4949). Retrieved June 2005 from U.S. National Institute for Deafness and other Communication Disorders Web site, under Health Information: http//:222.nidcd.nih.gov

National Network for Child Care. (2010). Better kid care: Play is the business of kids. Accessed January 24, 2010, from http://www.nncc.org/Curriculum/better.play.html

National Reading Panel (NRP). (2000). *Teaching children to read: An evidence-based assessment of the scientific research literature on reading and its implications for reading instruction: Report of the subgroups* (NIH Publication No. 00-4754). Washington, DC: National Institutes of Health and National Institute of Child Health and Human Development.

Nelson, N. W. (1990). *Planning individualized speech and language intervention programs.* Tucson, AZ: Communication Skill Builders.

Nelson, N. W. (2010). *Language and literacy disorders: Infancy through adolescence.* Boston, MA: Allyn-Bacon-Pearson.

Nelson, N. W., & Gillespie, L. L. (1991). *Analogies for thinking and talking: Words, pictures, and figures.* Tucson, AZ: Communication Skill Builders.

Neuman, S. B. (2004). *Introducing children to the world of writing.* Retrieved September 2009, from http://www2.scholastic.com/browse/article.jsp?id=3747261

Norbury, C., & Bishop, D. (2003). Narrative skills of children with communication impairments. *International Journal of Language and Communication Disorders, 38*(3), 287–313.

Numeroff, L. J. (1985). *If you give a mouse a cookie.* New York, NY: HarperCollins.

Nwakeze, P. C., & Seiler, L. H. (1993). Adult literacy programs: What students say. *Adult Learning, 5*, 17–18, 24.

O'Connor, J. (2007). *Fancy Nancy and the posh puppy.* New York, NY: HarperCollins.

Owens, R. E. (2010). *Language disorders: A functional approach to assessment and intervention.* Boston, MA: Pearson.

Pandell, K. (2006). *Peekaboo, stretch!* Cambridge, MA: Candlewick Press.

Parrot, K. (2008). *The link between art and literacy: The 5 stages of scribbling.* Retrieved September 15, 2009, from http://www.darienlibrary.org/node/1039

Paterson, D. (1981). *Stone soup.* Mahwah, NJ: Troll Associates.

Paul, R. (2001). *Language disorders from infancy through adolescence* (2nd ed.). St. Louis, MO: Mosby.

Paul, R. (2007). *Language disorders from infancy through adolescence* (3rd ed.). St. Louis, MO: Mosby.

Paul, R., & Smith, R. L. (1993). Narrative skills in 4-year-olds with normal, impaired, and late-developing language. *Journal of Speech and Hearing Disorders, 36,* 592–598.

Pepper, J., & Weitzman, E. (2004). *It takes two to talk* (3rd ed.). Toronto, Ontario: The Hanen Centre.

Pieretti, R. A. (2001). *Double-deficit reading disorders: A bottom-up perspective.* Unpublished master's thesis. California State University, Sacramento.

Powell, R., & Jones, K. (2002a). *Are you there, bunny?* Somerset, UK: Treehouse Childrens Books.

Powell, R., & Jones, K. (2002b). *I'll find you, kitty!* Somerset, UK: Treehouse Children's Books.

Powell, R., & Jones, K. (2002c). *Out you come, mouse!* Somerset, UK: Treehouse Children's Books.

Prifitera, A., Saklofske, D. A., & Weiss, L. G. (2004). *WISC- IV Clinical use and interpretation: Scientist-practitioner perspectives.* New York, NY: Elsevier.

Reading is Fundamental. (2009). Retrieved September 30, 2009, from http://www.rif.org

Reber, A. (1996). *Implicit learning.* Retrieved August 29, 2009, from http://74.125.45.132/search?q=cache:q5DCsorve-c]:www.spsp.org/student/intro/demos/implicit.doc+implicitlearning+cd

Richard, G. (2007). Language processing versus auditory processing. In D. S. Geffner & D. Ross-Swain (Eds.), *Auditory processing disorders: Assessment, management, and treatment* (pp. 161–174). San Diego, CA: Plural Publishing.

Rosen, M. (1989). *We're going on a bear hunt.* New York, NY: Margaret K. McElderry Books.

Rosner, J. (1987). *Green readiness book: Auditory and general activities for reading and arithmetic.* New York, NY: Walker and Company.

Rosner, J. (1993). *Helping children overcome learning difficulties* (3rd ed.). New York, NY: Walker and Company.

Rosner, M (2003). *We're going on a bear hunt.* New York, NY: Aladdin Paperbacks.

Ross-Swain, D. (2007). The speech-language pathologist's assessment of auditory processing disorders. In D. S. Geffner & D. Ross-Swain (Eds.),

Auditory processing disorders: Assessment, management, and treatment (pp. 139–174). San Diego, CA: Plural Publishing.

Ross-Swain, D, & Geffner, D. (2008, April). *Central auditory processing disorder: Assessment, management and treatment.* Presented at California Speech-Language-Hearing Annual State Conference, Monterey, CA.

Sandford, J. A. (1999–2001). *Soundsmart.* Richmond, VA: Braintrain.

Saracho, O., & Spodek, B. (2006). Young children's literacy-related play. *Early Child Development and Care, 176*(7), 707–721.

Sarback, S. (2008). Personal communication. Sacramento, CA.

Schwartz, S., & Miller, J. E. (1996). *The new language of toys: Teaching communication skills to children with special needs.* Bethesda. MD: Woodbine House.

Scott, C. (2004) Syntactic ability in children and adolescents with language and learning disabilities. In R. Berman (Ed.). *Language development across childhood and adolescence* (pp. 111–134). Philadelphia, PA: John Benjamin Publishing.

Scotton, R. (2008). *Splat the cat.* New York, NY: HarperCollins.

Semel, E., Wiig, E. H., & Secord, W. A. (2003). *Clinical evaluation of language fundamentals* (4th ed.). San Antonio, TX: PsychCorp.

Shipley, K. G., & McAfee, J. G. (2004). *Assessment in speech-language pathology: A resource manual* (3rd ed.). Clifton, Park, NY: Delmar Learning.

Sloan, C. (1986). *Treating auditory processing difficulties in children.* San Diego, CA: College-Hill Press.

Smilkstein, R. (2002). *We're born to learn: Using the brain's natural learning process to create today's curriculum.* Thousand Oaks, CA: Corwin Press.

Smilkstein, R. (2003). *The natural human learning process: Guidelines for curriculum development and lesson planning.* Available from http://www.borntolearn.net/pdf/guidelines.pdf

Snowling, M. J., Bishop, D. V. M., & Stothard, S. E, (2000). Is preschool language impairment at risk factor for dyslexia in adolescence? *Journal of Child Psychology and Psychiatry and Allied Disciplines, 41*(5), 587–600.

Speidel, G. E. (1993). Phonological short-term memory and individual differences in learning to speak: A bilingual case study. *First Language, 13*, 63–69.

Spitler-Kashuba, A. (2009). *A multimodal approach to narrative development.* Master's project, California State University, Sacramento, CA.

Stein, N., & Glenn C. (1979). An analysis of story comprehension in elementary school children. In R. D. Freedie (Ed.), *Advances in discourse processes. Vol 2: New directions in discourse processing* (pp. 53–119). Norwood, NJ: Ablex.

Tallal, P., Stark, R., & Mellits, D. (1985). The relationship between auditory temporal analysis and receptive language development: Evidence from studies of developmental language disorders. *Neuropsychologia, 23,* 527–534.

The nature of children's play. Avalable from http://www.kidsource.com/kidsource/content2.of.Nature.of.Childs.play.html

Think It Through Tiles. (1979). Livermore, CA: Discovery Toys.

Thompson, R. (1990). *Draw-and-tell.* Toronto, Ontario: Annick Press Ltd.

Torgesen, J. K., & Mathes, P. G. (2000). *A basic guide to understanding, assessing, and teaching phonological awareness.* Austin, TX: Pro-Ed.

Turk, H. (1981). *Max.* Neugebauer Press distributed in Natick, MA: by Alphabet Press.

Turk, H. (1984a). *Happy birthday Max.* Boston, MA: Neugebauer Press.

Turk, H. (1984b). *Max packs.* Boston, MA: Neugebauer Press.

Tyler, A., Edwards, M. L., & Saxman, J. H. (1987). Clinical application of two phonologically based treatment procedures. *Journal of Speech and Hearing Disorders, 52,* 393–409.

Ultimate phonics [Software]. (2000). San Diego, CA: Spencer Learning.

UpWords [Game]. (1997) New York, NY: Milton Bradley Company.

Wagner, R., Torgesen, J., & Rashotte, C. (1999). *Comprehensive test of phonological processing.* San Antonio, TX: Pearson.

Wallach, G. P., & Miller, L. (1988). *Language intervention and academic success.* San Diego, CA: College-Hill Press/Little Brown.

Watkins, C. & Kadem, F. (1994). Neurobiology of specific language impairment: Future research. *Brain Research, 64,* 213–218.

Watson, C. (1983). *Aesop's fables.* London, UK: Usborne Publishing Ltd.

Webster's new world college dictionary. (2002). Somerset, NJ: Wiley.

West, T. G. (1997). *In the mind's eye.* Amherst, NY: Prometheus Books.

West, T. G. (2008, Summer). It is time to get serious about the talents of dyslexics. *Perspectives on Language and Literacy, 34*(3), 9–11.

Westby, C. (2000). A scale for assessing development of children's play. In K. Gitlin-Weiner, A. Sandgund, & C. Schaefer (Eds.), *Play diagnostic and assessment* (pp. 15–57). New York, NY: Wiley.

Westby, C., & McKellar, N. (2000). Autism. In E. P. Dodge (Ed.), *The survival guide for school-based speech-language pathologists* (pp. 263–303). Clifton Park, NY: Delmar Learning.

Wilson, C., Lanza, J. R., & Evans, J. S. (2005). *Revised SLP IEP companion.* East Moline, IL: LinguiSystems.

Wolf, M., Miller, L., & Donnelly, K. (2000). Retrieval, automaticity, vocabulary elaboration, orthography (RAVE-O). *Journal of Learning Disabilities, 33,* 375–386.

Wood, A. (1984). *The napping house.* New York, NY: Harcourt Brace Jovanovich.

Wood, A., & Wood, B. (2003). *Alphabet mystery.* New York, NY: The Blue Sky Press.

Woodcock, R. J., McGrew, K. W., & Mather, N. (2007). *Woodcock-Johnson III.* Rolling Meadows, IL: Riverside Publishing.

Word families with silly sentences. (2004). Greenville, SC: SuperDuper Publications.

Woodcock, R. W. (1991).*Woodcock Language Proficiency Battery-Revised* (WLPB-R). Allen, TX: DLM Teaching Resources.

Word families with silly sentences. (2004). Greenville, SC: SuperDuper Publications.

Zimmerman, I, L., Steiner, V. G., & Pond, R. E. (2002). *Preschool language scale* (4th ed.) San Antonio, TX: PsychCorp.

Index